Manual on *Shirish Sheth* VAGINAL SURGERY

Manual on *Shirish Sheth* VAGINAL SURGERY

Series Editors

Nandita Palshetkar
MD FCPS FICOG FRCOG (UK)
Professor Emeritus
Department of Obstetrics and Gynecology
DY Patil School of Medicine
Navi Mumbai, Maharashtra, India
Founder and Medical Director of the
Famous Bloom IVF Group

Hrishikesh D Pai
MD FRCOG (UK-HON) FCPS FICOG MSc (USA)
Trustee, FIGO, Asia Oceania (2023–25)
Professor, DY Patil University
Navi Mumbai, Maharashtra, India
Immediate Past President FOGSI (2022–23)
Founder and Medical Director
Bloom IVF Group, Mumbai

Niranjan Chavan
MD FICOG FCPS DGO DFP MICOG DICOG Diploma in Endoscopy (USA)
Professor and Unit Chief
Department of Obstetrics and Gynecology
Lokmanya Tilak Medical College and General Hospital
Mumbai, Maharashtra, India

Editors

Rajendra Saraogi
MD FCPS FICOG DGO
Emirates Professor, Seth GS Medical College
Retired Hon and HOD, Cooper Hospital
Senior Consultant
Max Nanavati Hospital
Mumbai, Maharashtra, India
Director Saraogi Group of Hospitals

Suman Sinha
MBBS DGO FICOG FIAOG FIAMS
Senior Consultant
Department of Obstetric and Gynecology
AH IVF and Research Center
Ranchi, Jharkhand, India

Kanchan Sharma MBBS MS FICOG FICMCH
Director and Senior Consultant
Aakash IVF, Kanpur, Uttar Pradesh, India
Chairperson of Noncommunicable Disease Committee FOGSI

Co-Editors

PC Mahapatra, Hara Pattanaik, Mohit Saraogi
Anuja Pawde, Jagruti Ghosh

JAYPEE BROTHERS MEDICAL PUBLISHERS
The Health Sciences Publisher
New Delhi | London

Message from Series Editors

Dear AICOG 2025 delegates,

It is a matter of great pride that the landmark AICOG 2025 is being held in the city of Mumbai, Maharashtra, India. The Organizing Committee and the hosts Mumbai Obstetric and Gynaecological Society have left no stone unturned in their quest to make this a historic event by aiming to have a scientific program of the highest caliber, punctuated by fantastic keynotes and orations, graced by the best international faculty in the field of Obstetrics, Gynecology and its subspecialities along with a cultural treat every evening to cater to the audience which hails from far-flung corners of India and the globe.

On this occasion, the academic stalwarts and senior FOGSIans have burned the midnight oil at both ends to contribute and create a set of AICOG 2025 Workshop Manuals that aim to amalgamate the most recent scientific advancements and evidence-based best practices in a nutshell for the delegates to take home and implement in their practices when they have returned from this magnificent event.

We acknowledge the efforts of all the editors, co-editors, authors, co-authors, co-contributors and junior authors who have sometimes worked at short notice to submit excellent chapters and articles included in the final publication. We also wish to take this opportunity to thank Shri Jitendar P Vij (Group Chairman) and Mr Ankit Vij (Managing Director) of M/s Jaypee Brothers Medical Publishers (P) Ltd, New Delhi, India, in publishing the book and their associates, particularly Ms Chetna Malhotra (Senior Director—Professional Publishing, Marketing, and Business Development), Ms Kritika Dua (Senior Commissiong Editor), and Mr Priyansh Saxena (Development Editor), who have been prompt, efficient, and most helpful.

We hope that the delegates and the attendees will enjoy reading this publication and the scientific data included therein will help to shape your knowledge, attitudes and practices and ultimately benefit the women of our country, whom we all serve.

Nandita Palshetkar
Organizing Chairperson, AICOG Mumbai, 2025

Hrishikesh D Pai
Chairperson, Scientific Committee, AICOG Mumbai, 2025

Niranjan Chavan
Organizing Secretary, AICOG Mumbai, 2025

FOGSI

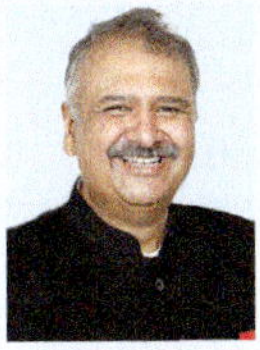

Jaydeep Tank
President 2024–2025

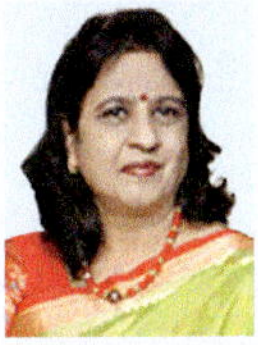

Madhuri Patel
Secretary General

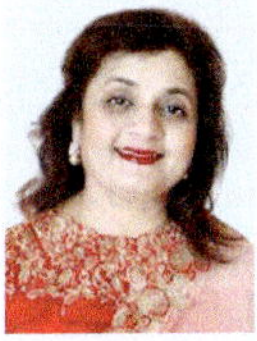

Sunita Tandulwadkar
President 2025–2026

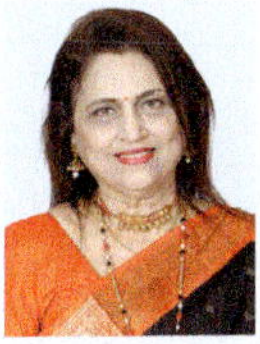

Suvarna Khadilkar
Deputy Secretary General

AICOG 2025 Core Committee

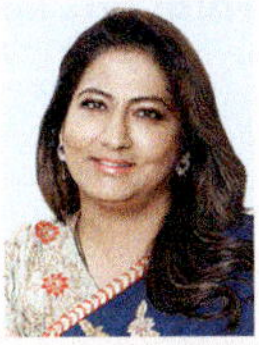

Nandita Palshetkar
Organizing Chairperson

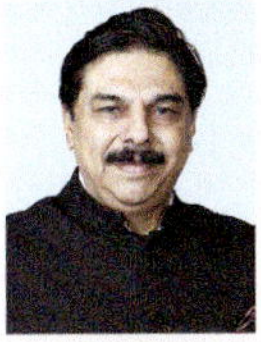

Hrishikesh D Pai
Chairperson, Scientific Committee

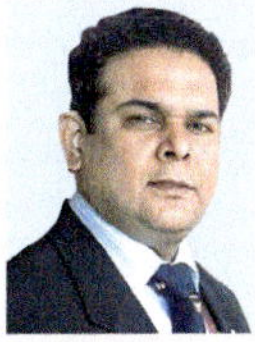

Niranjan Chavan
Organizing Secretary

Editors

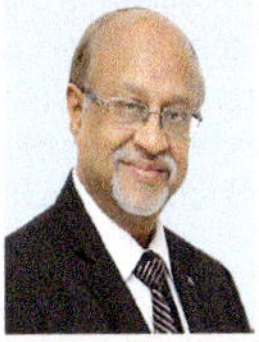

Rajendra Saraogi

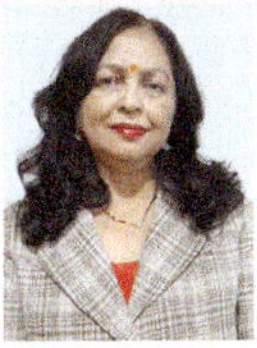

Suman Sinha

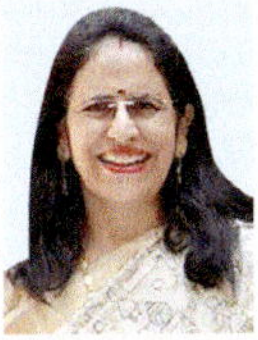

Kanchan Sharma

Vice Chairpersons

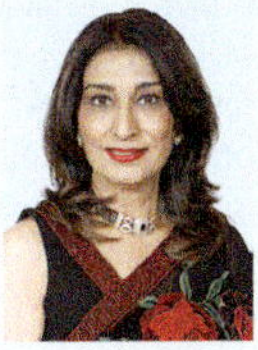

Rishma Dhillon Pai

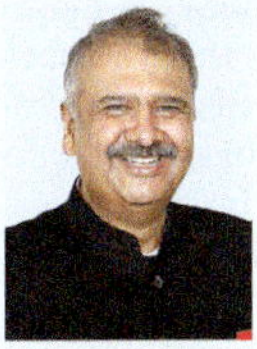

Jaydeep Tank

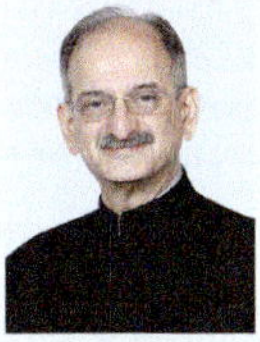

Nozer Sheriar

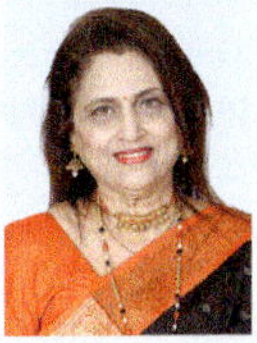

Suvarna Khadilkar

AICOG 2025 Publication Committee

Pratik Tambe | **Rohan Palshetkar**
Pradnya Supe | **Manan Boob**

Jaypee Brothers Medical Publishers (P) Ltd

Headquarters
EMCA House
23/23-B, Ansari Road, Daryaganj
New Delhi 110 002, India
Landline: +91-11-23272143, +91-11-23272703
+91-11-23282021, +91-11-23245672
E-mail: jaypee@jaypeebrothers.com

Corporate Office
Jaypee Brothers Medical Publishers (P) Ltd.
4838/24, Ansari Road, Daryaganj
New Delhi 110 002, India
Phone: +91-11-43574357
Fax: +91-11-43574314
E-mail: jaypee@jaypeebrothers.com

Overseas Office
JP Medical Ltd.
83, Victoria Street, London
SW1H 0HW (UK)
Phone: +44-20 3170 8910
E-mail: info@jpmedpub.com

EU GPSR Authorised Representative Logos Europe, 9 rue Nicolas Poussin 17000, La Rochelle, France
Phone: +33 (0) 6 67 93 73 78
E-mail: Contact@logoseurope.eu

Website: www.jaypeebrothers.com
Website: www.jaypeedigital.com

Inquiries for bulk sales may be solicited at: jaypee@jaypeebrothers.com

Manual on Shirish Sheth Vaginal Surgery

First Edition: **2025**

ISBN: 978-93-6616-656-8

Printed in India

Contributors

Akash Gajjar
GO DNB FICOG Fellow in Clinical Embryology
Practising Obs - Gyne Since 10 Years and in IVF Practice Since 6 Years
Ashirwad Hospital (Chikhli) and Akash IVF Center (Navsari)
Gujarat, Ahemadabad, India

Anil Sakhare
MBBS DGO DNB DFP FICOG
Consultant
Department of Obstetrics and Gynecology
Rayat Hospital
Nanded, Maharashtra, India

Asavari Karani
MS FCPS (Gold Medalist)
Consultant
Tulshi Clinic and Holi Family Hospital
Mumbai, Maharashtra, India

Ashok Kumar Todani
MBBS DGO FICOG FICMU Diploma in Surgical Pelviscopy (Kiel, Germany)
Director
Sonography Clinic and Laparoscopy Center
Raniganj, West Bengal, India
Attached to MRS Hospital
Lions Nursing Home
BN Agarwal Hospital
Subhdarshini Multi-speciality Hospital

Kanchan Sharma
MBBS MS FICOG FICMCH
Director and Senior Consultant
Aakash IVF
Kanpur, Uttar Pradesh, India
Chairperson of Noncommunicable Disease Committee FOGSI

Kartikeya Bhagat MD FICOG IBCLC
Director
Grace Maternity and Nursing Home, Kandivali West
Mumbai, Maharashtra, India

Kiran Lata Todani
MBBS DA
Director
Sonography Clinic and Laparoscopy Center
Raniganj, West Bengal, India
Attached to MRS Hospital
Lions Nursing Home
BN Agarwal Hospital
Subhdarshini Multi-speciality Hospital

Manohar Motwani
MD DGO FCPS
Honorary Rajawadi Hospital, Mumbai
Director Karbhari Nursing Home, Mumbai
Consultant Surya Hospital
Criticare Hospital
Mumbai, Maharashtra, India

Mohan A Gadam
MD DGO DFP FICS FICOG DNBE GOLD MEDAL AT DFP and DGO
Postgraduate Teacher
University of Mumbai
Ex Associate Professor
LTMG Hospital and LTMMC, Mumbai
Ex HOD Dr RN Cooper Hospital, Mumbai
Vice President Maharashtra Chapter SOVSI

Monika Anant
MBBS MS FICOG FMAS
Professor
Department of Obstetrics and Gynecology
All India Institute of Medical Sciences
Patna, Bihar, India

Monika Dalal
MD
Professor
PGIMS
Rohtak, Haryana, India

Mukesh Rathi
MD DNB DGO FCPS
Consultant Gynecologist
Vaginal Surgeon and Obstetrician
Akola, Maharashtra, India

Narendra D Gajjar
DGO MD
Practicing Obstetrician and Gynecologist
Ashirwad Hospital (Chikhli) and Akash IVF Center, Navsari
Gujarat, Ahemadabad, India

Niharika Allu
MS (Obs & Gyne) DNB FICOG
Consultant Obstetrician and Gynecologist
Rainbow Children's Hospital and Birthright
Visakhapatnam, Andhra Pradesh, India

Nilakshi Phukan Kumar
MBBS MD (Obs & Gyne)
Senior Consultant
Down Town Hospital
Director Gynec Center (Women and Fertility Clinic)
Guwahati, Assam, India

Pankaj Sarode
MBBS MD
Director
Cradle Maternity and Women Care, Pune
Head
Department of Vaginal Reconstruction and Cosmetic Gynecology
Ankura Hospital
Pune, Maharashtra, India

Partha Sarathi Tripathy
MBBS FCGP
Assistant Professor
MKCG Medical College and Hospital
Berhampur, Odisha, India

Punam Dixit
MBBS (Honors) MS MRCOG (London) FRCOG (London)
Consultant
Punam Surgical and Maternity Hospital
Patna, Bihar, India

Ragini Agrawal
MS
Director
A A Dermascience "Complete Clinic for Women's Health"
Gurugram, Haryana, India

Rajendra Saraogi
MD FCPS FICOG DGO
Emirates Professor
Seth GS Medical College
Retired Hon and HOD
Cooper Hospital
Senior Consultant
Max Nanavati Hospital
Mumbai, Maharashtra, India
Director Saraogi Group of Hospitals

Rajeshree Jain
MBBS MS (Obs & Gyne)
Senior Consultant
Max Hospital
New Delhi, India

Rajkumar H Shah
MD FCPS FICS FICOG DGO DFP
Senior Consultant Gynecologist
Nanavati Max Super Specialty Hospital
Med Director, Eva Medicare Pvt Ltd
President, Association of Fellow Gynecologists
Mumbai, Maharashtra, India

Richa Narkhade
MBBS MS FMAS Dip in Urogynecology
Assistant Professor
SAIMS
Indore, Madhya Pradesh, India

Samir R Pradhan
MD DNB FCPS DGO DFP
Proprietor: Samarth Maternity and Nursing Home, Mumbai
Consultant
Department of Obstetrics and Gynecology
Godrej Memorial Hospital
Vikhroli, Mumbai, Maharashtra
Fortis Hospital
Jupiter Hospital
Thane, Maharashtra, India

Sandhya Rani Panigrahy
MD OG FICOG MICOG FICMCH FCGP FIAOG FMAS CPIMS MWPM
OG Consultant, Addl Director
Practicing Gynecologist
Gayatri Hospital
Berhampur, Odisha, India

Sonam Kataria
MS DNB
Consultant
RMS Multispecialty Hospital
Kandivali West, Maharashtra, India

Sucheta Hiray-Bachhav
MD DGO
Director
Tulshi Multispecialty Hospital
Visiting Consultant
Sahyadri Hospital
Nashik, Maharashtra, India

Suman Sinha
MBBS DGO FICOG FIAOG FIAMS
Senior Consultant
Department of Obstetric and Gynecology
AH IVF and Research Center
Ranchi, Jharkhand, India

T Srikala Prasad
MD DGO MCh (Urology)
Professor and Head
Department of Urology
Government Kilpauk Medical College
Chennai, Tamil Nadu, India

Uma Rani Swain
MD (Obs & Gyne)
Senior Director
BLK-Max Super Speciality Hospital
New Delhi, India

Preface

The updated manual on *Shirish Sheth Vaginal Surgery* by FOGSI, features 21 comprehensive chapters that embodies the entire spectrum of vaginal surgeries right from understanding the anatomy of the vagina and case selection to postoperative care. It has been presented in a very crisp and concise manner with the sole purpose of imparting basics and fundamental knowledge to enhance the surgical skills of practicing doctors and students.

The authors have dedicated countless hours in meticulously compiling the chapters. We are immensely thankful to them.

We are equally obliged and grateful to our leaders of FOGSI Dr Hrishikesh D Pai, Dr Rishma Pai, Dr Nandita Palshetkar, Dr Niranjan Chavan and Dr Rohan Palshetkar for believing in us and giving us the opportunity. We are indebted to them for their unwavering support and guidance.

Our sincere thanks to Shri Jitendar P Vij (Group Chairman) and Mr Ankit Vij (Managing Director) of M/s Jaypee Brothers Medical Publishers (P) Ltd New Delhi, India for their support, encouragement and logistics. We express our special thanks to the entire production team of M/s Jaypee Brothers Medical Publishers (P) Ltd especially, Mr Priyansh Saxena (Development Editor) for their hard work, professionalism and for helping us throughout the journey of this publication.

May the manual be a guiding light to serve as a invaluable resources in understanding the intricacies of vaginal surgeries for our practitioners and academicians.

"If you have knowledge, Let the others light their candles in it"

Happy reading to our Readers

Series Editors: Nandita Palshetkar, Hrishikesh D Pai, Niranjan Chavan
Editors: Rajendra Saraogi, Suman Sinha, Kanchan Sharma
Co-Editors: PC Mahapatra, Hara Pattanaik, Mohit Saraogi, Anuja Pawde, Jagruti Ghosh

Contents

1 CHAPTER

Understanding the Anatomy of the Vagina: A Comprehensive Guide

Ragini Agrawal, Monika Dalal

INTRODUCTION

Vagina is the cornerstone of the female reproductive system, embodying both complexity and resilience. Its structural integrity and functionality are supported by a multifaceted network of anatomical components. By comprehensively understanding the anatomy and function of vaginal support, we aim to shed light on the importance of this intricate system in women's health and well-being.

Functions of vagina are passage for sexual intercourse, transport of sperms, expulsion of the menstrual blood and the delivery of the baby. It is a narrow, muscular but elastic organ and connects the external genital organs to the uterus. It starts at the vulva externally and ends at the cervix internally. The posterior wall is about 4.5 inches long, whereas the anterior wall is about 3.5 inches.[1] Therefore, the posterior vaginal wall is longer than the anterior vaginal wall. In relaxing position, the anterior and posterior walls of vagina are in contact with each other.

The vaginal portion of the cervix protrudes into the upper anterior part of the vagina, which leads to the formation of anterior, posterior, and lateral fornices. As cervix protrudes through anterior vagina, posterior fornix is the deepest.

There are three sulci on the anterior vaginal wall. Submeatal sulcus lies above the urethral meatus. There is another sulcus, about 3.5 cm above submeatal sulcus in the anterior vaginal wall, called as transverse vaginal sulcus. It corresponds to the junction of urethra and bladder. Further above is the sulcus of bladder and indicates the junction of the bladder to the anterior vaginal wall.

G-Spot: The Grafenberg spot, commonly known as the G-spot, is an erogenous zone located on the anterior wall of the vagina, about 1–2 inches from the entrance. Stimulation of the G-spot can lead to intense sexual pleasure and, for some individuals, orgasm.[2]

Epithelium: The vaginal mucosa is lined by stratified squamous epithelium. There are no glands in the vagina and the vaginal secretions are mainly derived from the mucus discharge of the cervix and transudation through the vaginal epithelium. The vestibular glands located in labia minora provide moisture for the vagina. Normal pH of vagina during reproductive age is about 4.5. Acidic pH inhibits the growth of other pathogenic organisms and increases resistance to infection.

RELATIONS (FIG. 1)

Anterior: Anteriorly, the vagina is related to the bladder in upper two-thirds and urethra in the lower third. It is not covered with peritoneum anteriorly.

Posterior: Posteriorly, vagina is related to the rectouterine pouch (pouch of Douglas), the ampulla of rectum, the perineal body, and the anal canal.

Lateral: Ureter, uterine artery, levator ani muscle, and the urogenital diaphragm.

Blood Supply

The blood supply of vagina is by the vaginal and uterine branches of the internal iliac artery. Inferior vesical and middle rectal arteries anastomose freely on the vaginal wall and also contribute to the blood supply of vagina. The venous drainage of vagina is through the vaginal venous plexus with the vaginal vein which drains into the internal iliac vein or the uterine vein.

Nerve Supply

The uterovaginal nerve plexus lying in the base of the broad ligament gives rise to the parasympathetic and sympathetic nerves supplying the vagina. The sympathetic fibers are derived from lumbar splanchnic nerves, whereas

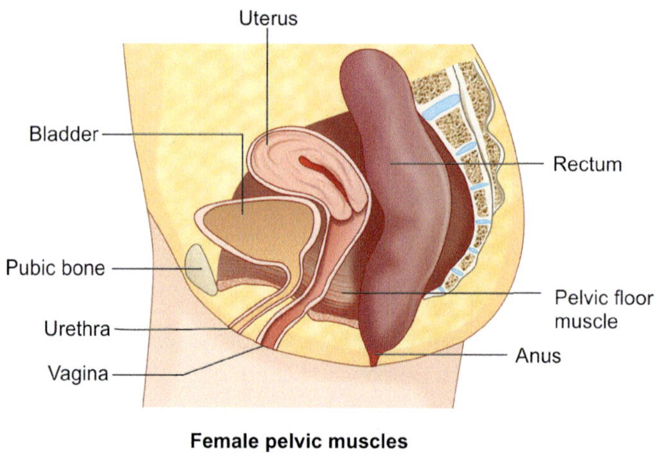

Fig. 1: Relations of vagina.

the parasympathetic fibers are derived from the pelvic splanchnic nerves. The nerve supply to the lower part of the vagina is from the branch of pudendal nerve called the deep perineal nerve.

Lymphatic Drainage

The lower one-third of the vagina drains to the superficial inguinal lymph nodes (similar to the vulval drainage), while the upper two-thirds drain into the external and internal iliac and sacral nodes (similar to that of cervix).

Supports of Vagina

If one looks at the vaginal canal from the side, he or she can appreciate different levels of support as described by DeLancey and colleagues.[3]

Level I: Uterosacral and cardinal ligaments

Level II: Levator ani

Level III: Perineal membrane

Level I: Uterosacral and Cardinal Ligaments

The level I support is composed of the uterosacral and cardinal ligaments that form the support of the uterus and upper one-third of the vagina **(Fig. 2)**. In level I, the paracolpium connects the vagina from the lateral pelvic walls. Fibers of level I extend both vertically and also posteriorly toward the sacrum.

Clinical significance: The upper portions of the anterior vaginal wall can prolapse due to lack of level I support and failure of uterosacral-cardinal complex. With time, this may increase load in the paravaginal area and lead to failure of Level II paravaginal support. Resuspension of the vaginal apex

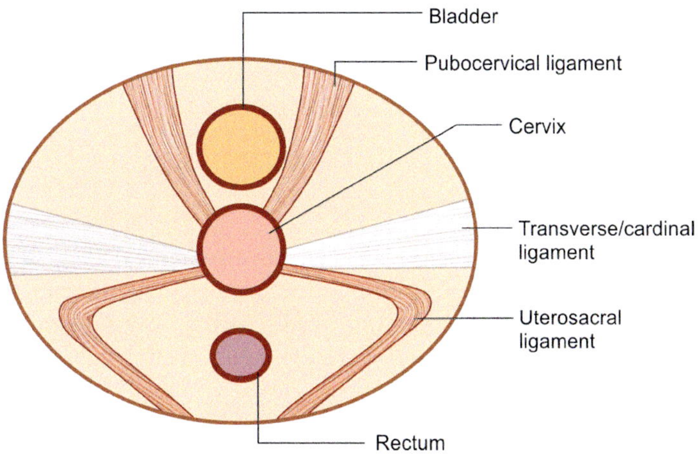

Fig. 2: Uterosacral and cardinal ligaments.

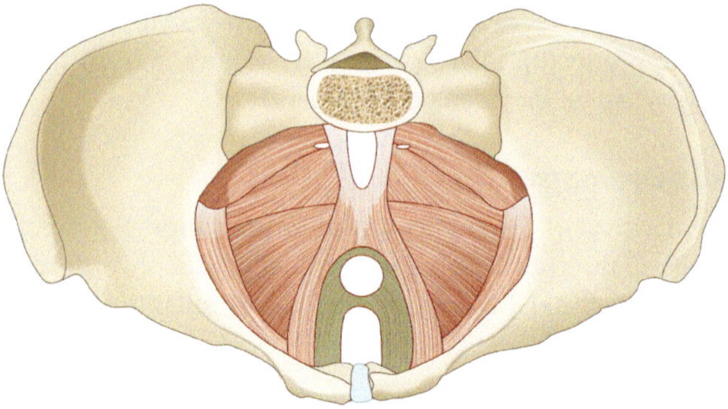

Fig. 3: Levator ani muscle.

at the time of surgery, in addition to paravaginal or anterior colporrhaphy, may help to return the anterior wall to a more normal position or at least to prevent future failures.[4]

Level II: Levator Ani

It is the most important muscle in the pelvic floor. It has slow-twitch fibers which maintain a constant tone and fast-twitch (type II) fibers with an increased density in the periurethral and perianal areas. The levator ani muscle is in a continuous state of contraction, similar to the external anal sphincter and some postural muscles and keeps the urogenital hiatus closed by compressing the urethra, vagina, and rectum towards the pubic bone.

Attachment: Levator ani **(Fig. 3)** is attached to posterior surface of pubis, fascia over obturator internus called arcus tendineus and ischial spine and inserts on coccyx and then meets in the midline on the midline raphe. Arcus tendineus is a fascial thickening on the surface of obturator internus muscle bilaterally that runs from the pubic ramus ventrally to the ischial spine dorsally and gives origin to levator ani.

The levator ani comprised of three striated muscles:

1. Puborectalis
2. Pubococcygeus
3. Ileococcygeus

Puborectalis muscle: These are the thicker, narrower medial fibers of levator ani muscle **(Fig. 4)**. Its origin is from posterior aspects of the right and left pubic bones. It passes inferiorly to fuse with its opposite side and form a U-shaped sling behind the ano-rectum and bounds the urogenital hiatus.

Pubococcygeus muscle: These are the intermediate fibers of levator ani which is lateral to puborectalis **(Fig. 5)**. It originates from the inner surface of the pubic bone and arcus tendineus and passes posteriorly. Medial fibers merge

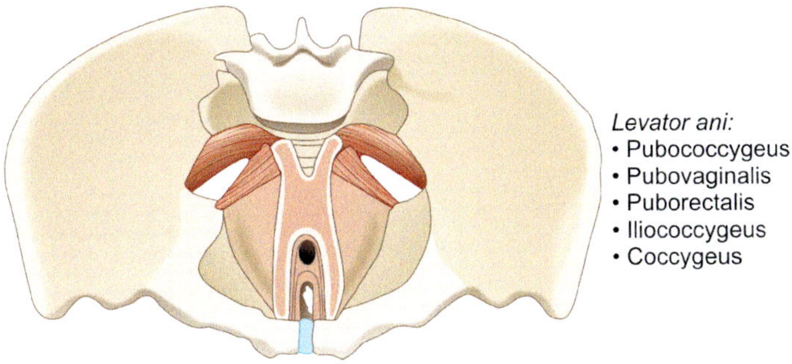

Fig. 4: Puborectalis muscle.

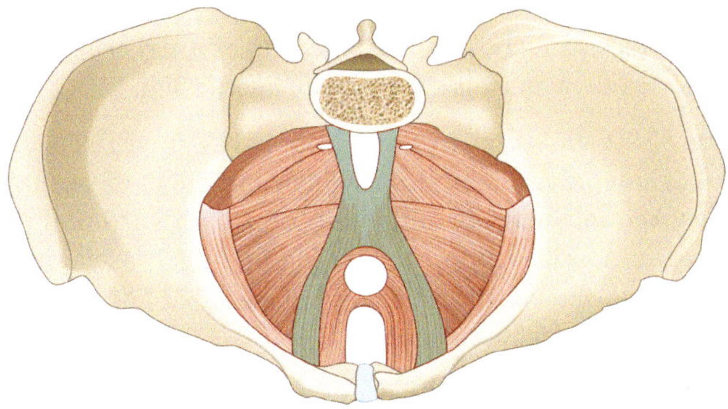

Fig. 5: Pubococcygeus muscle.

with fibers from opposite side and form levator plate and anococcygeal raphe. It loops around vagina and anorectal portions and insert into perineal body and external anal sphincter muscle. The urethral part merges with the periuretheral musculature.

Ileococcygeus: They are the thin posterolateral fibers of levator ani **(Fig. 6)**. It originates from posterior tendinous arc and ischial spine. Posteriorly, the medial fibers merge to form levator plate and lateral fibers insert to the last two segments of the coccyx.

Levator plate: Medial fibers of the opposite sides of levator ani merge together behind the anus and form a fibrous raphe or tendinous plate called levator plate which is between anus and the coccyx. It provides a shelf on which the pelvic organs like uterus, upper vagina, and rectum rest. The levator plate is horizontal in standing position.

Urogenital hiatus: In the midline anteriorly, levator ani muscle has a U-shaped defect called urogenital hiatus which gives passage to the urethra and vagina. It is supported anteriorly by pubic bones, the levator ani muscles laterally,

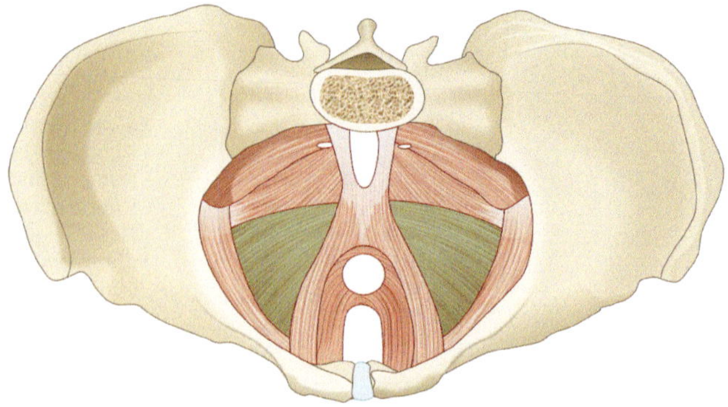

Fig. 6: Ileococcygeus muscle.

and dorsally (posteriorly) by perineal body and external anal sphincter. The perineal membrane covers this gap from the inferior side.

Fascia: The Silent Architect: Wrapping the pelvic floor like a supportive sheath, fascia emerges as an indispensable component of vaginal support, providing structural integrity and cohesion to the surrounding tissues. Several layers of fascia—endopelvic fascia, perineal fascia, and visceral pelvic fascia—contribute to the robustness of the pelvic floor and its ability to withstand intra-abdominal pressure.[5]

Clinical significance: Level I and levator ani muscles are interdependent. Intact levator ani muscles balance the tension of the level I support structures, and intact level I support lessens the pressure imposed from above on the pelvic floor.

In level II, the vagina gets its support by levator ani, arcus tendineus fasciae pelvis and the superior fascia of levator ani. Anterior vaginal wall, through its connections to the arcus tendineus fascia pelvis, forms a supportive layer clinically referred to as the pubocervical fascia. A simple case of a distension cystocele could result from a defect in pubocervical fibromuscularis. Detachment of arcus tendineus from the levator ani is associated with stress incontinence and anterior prolapse. The detachment can be unilateral or bilateral, causing a displacement cystocele.[6]

As in the anterior compartment, a simple defect in rectovaginal fibromuscularis can cause a distention rectocele. A defect in the posterior arcus also called arcus tendineus rectovaginalis (ATRV) is associated with a pararectal defect that can be unilateral or bilateral.

Level III: The Perineal Membrane

A critical but perhaps underappreciated part of the pelvic floor support is the perineal membrane as it forms level III support **(Fig. 7)**. It is a single connective tissue membrane, with muscle lying immediately above. The

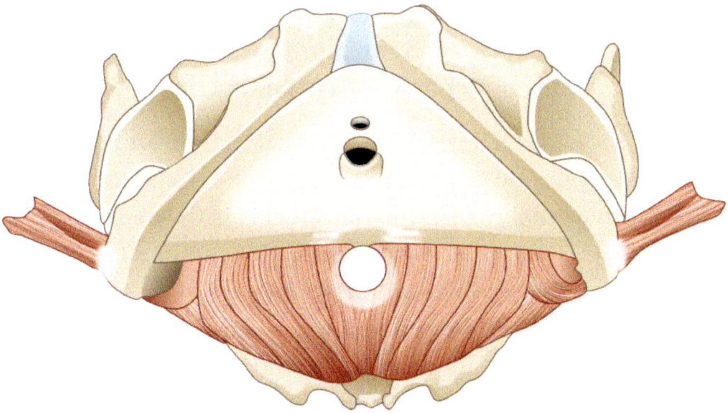

Fig. 7: Perineal membrane.

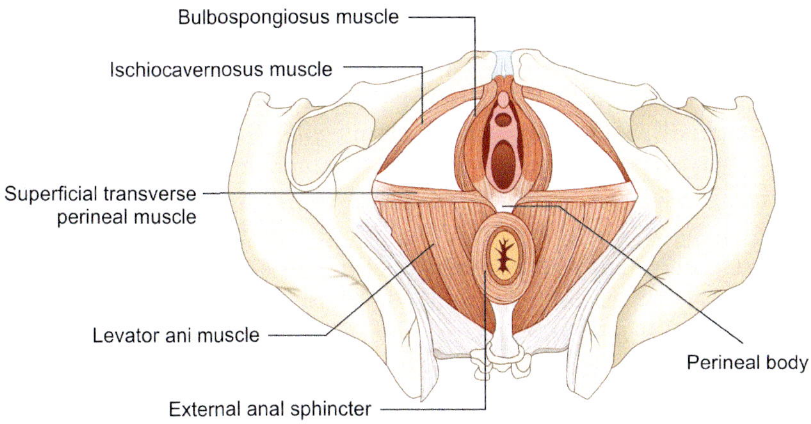

Fig. 8: Perineal body.

perineal membrane is at the level of the hymen, and it gives support to vagina by attaching it to perineal body and ischiopubic rami.

It lies inferior to the urogenital hiatus of the levator ani muscle. It is a triangular sheet of dense, fibromuscular tissue that spans the anterior half of the pelvic outlet and is attached to the bony framework of a pubic arch. It has two openings, for urethra and vagina.

Perineal body: Perineal body is also called central tendon of the perineum. It is ill-defined connective tissue structure and lies at the midpoint of posterior border of perineal membrane **(Fig. 8)**. It is bound anteriorly by the lower vagina, posteriorly by anus and below by perineal skin. Occupying a central position within the perineum, the perineal body emerges as a nexus of connective tissue and muscle, orchestrating the symphony of pelvic support. This fibromuscular structure serves as a convergence point for various muscles and ligaments, including the levator ani, transverse perineal muscle, and superficial perineal muscles. By anchoring these structures to a common focal point, the perineal body contributes to pelvic floor stability and function

Clinical significance: The fibers of the perineal membrane connect through the perineal body, thereby providing a layer that resists downward descent of the rectum. If perineal membrane support is lost, then the resistance to downward descent is lost and a perineocele develops.[7] Clinical diagnosis of this can be made by realizing the patient's need to splint close to the vaginal opening to have a bowel movement, and on physical examination an elongated or "empty" perineal body can be noticed. During perineorrhaphy, reattachment of the separated structures can correct this defect and is a mainstay of reconstructive surgery.

CONCLUSION

The support of the vagina is an intricate tapestry woven from the threads of the uterosacral and cardinal ligaments, levator ani, endopelvic fascia, perineal membrane and perineal body. Each of these anatomical components plays a pivotal role in maintaining pelvic floor integrity, supporting pelvic organs, and facilitating normal pelvic function. Dysfunction or weakness within this complex system can manifest as pelvic floor disorders, including pelvic organ prolapse, urinary incontinence, or sexual dysfunction, necessitating targeted interventions to restore pelvic support and alleviate symptoms. By comprehensively understanding the anatomy and function of vaginal support, healthcare providers can tailor treatment strategies to address individual needs and optimize women's pelvic health and well-being. Moreover, promoting awareness and education about vaginal support empowers individuals to advocate for their own reproductive health and seek timely intervention when needed.

REFERENCES

1. Gold JM, Shrimanker I. Physiology, Vaginal. [Updated 2023 Jul 24]. In: StatPearls [Internet]. Treasure Island (FL): StatPearls Publishing; 2024 Jan-. Available from: https://www.ncbi.nlm.nih.gov/books/NBK545147/.
2. Ellibeş Kaya A, Çalışkan E. Women self-reported G-spot existence and relation with sexual function and genital perception. Turk J Obstet Gynecol. 2018;15(3):182-7. doi: 10.4274/tjod.55531. Epub 2018 Sep 3. PMID: 30202629; PMCID: PMC6127477.
3. DeLancey JO. Anatomic aspects of vaginal eversion after hysterectomy. Am J Obstet Gynecol. 1992;166(6 Pt 1):1717-24. [PubMed] [Google Scholar]
4. Arenholt LTS, Pedersen BG, Glavind K, Glavind-Kristensen M, DeLancey JOL. Paravaginal defect: anatomy, clinical findings, and imaging. Int Urogynecol J. 2017;28(5):661-73. doi: 10.1007/s00192-016-3096-3. Epub 2016 Sep 17. PMID: 27640064; PMCID: PMC5429977.

5. Roch M, Gaudreault N, Cyr MP, Venne G, Bureau NJ, Morin M. The female pelvic floor fascia anatomy: a systematic search and review. Life (Basel). 2021;11(9):900. doi: 10.3390/life11090900. PMID: 34575049; PMCID: PMC8467746.
6. Garg R, Malhotra J. Pelvic Organ Prolapse: From basics to newer evolutions in surgical management of uterine prolapse. J South Asian Feder Menopause Soc 2020;8(1):1-6.
7. Eilber KS, Rosenblum N, Gore J, Raz S, Rodríguez LV. Perineocele: symptom complex, description of anatomic defect, and surgical technique for repair. Urology. 2006;67(2):265-8. doi: 10.1016/j.urology.2005.08.060. Epub 2006 Jan 26. PMID: 16442600.

2 CHAPTER

Case Selection for Vaginal Hysterectomy

Narendra D Gajjar, Akash Gajjar

INTRODUCTION

Hysterectomy is the 2nd most common surgery on women during reproductive age, next to cesarean section. Once the decision of hysterectomy is taken, route of hysterectomy should be determined prior to surgery.

Vaginal hysterectomy is a minimally invasive procedure[1] it has distinct advantages over abdominal and total laparoscopic hysterectomy such as less operative time, minimal blood loss, minimal complications, minimal hospital stay, least post operative pain, very early post operative recovery, return to work and most cost effective so vaginal hysterectomy is preferred because of lower morbidity and quicker recovery when there is no contraindication.[2]

Case selection for vaginal hysterectomy is a crucial decision. It depends upon many factors including skill, experience and confidence of surgeon.

Patient should be examined by operating surgeon himself, so that assessment of all favoring factors as well as anticipation of difficulties can be predicted in advance. This helps surgeon to do meticulous planning and overcome these difficulties according to skill and experience with an open mind to change the course of surgery if needed.

COMMON INDICATIONS OF HYSTERECTOMY

It is a recommended intervention in a variety of gynecological conditions, including:[1] AUB, symptomatic fibroids endometriosis, adenomyosis, genital prolapse, pelvic inflammatory disease, uterine, cervical and ovarian malignancy.

- For every hysterectomy counseling is the most integral part. We should take in consideration various factors like age of patient, desire to preserve childbearing function and medical conditions.
- Various optional treatment modalities should be discussed in detail with patient and her relatives including its benefits and disadvantages.
- Choice should be on the part of the patient. Entire procedure including preoperative preparation, operative details and possible complications though rare should be explained.

Essential Factors for Planning Surgery

History taking, clinical examination and medical assessment are the most important factors. Points in history that may guide the route of hysterectomy.

- Age, parity and previous vaginal delivery
- Menstrual disorders
- Dysmenorrhea/pelvic pain
- Dyspareunia
- Lump arising from pelvis, heaviness
- Something coming out p/v and defects of pelvic floor including cystocele, enterocele, rectocele, urethrocele and relaxed vaginal opening with its associated symptoms
- Previous surgeries especially cesarean section or hysterotomy/laparotomy with single or multiple scars
- Symptoms suggestive of malignancy
- Pelvic pain or pain suggestive of adhesions, endometriosis.
- Strong family history of ca ovary, uterus or breast
- Obesity
- H/O allergy or anaphylaxis to drugs

PREOPERATIVE ASSESSMENT

- Patient should be clinically examined and evaluated by routine and if required specific investigations Cardiovascular, Respiratory and Neurological assessment should be done.
- CBC, Blood group, PP2BS, S. Creatinine, Urine R and M, SGPT, PT, APTT, INR, ECG and if suggested 2D echo and other specific investigations should be done. Preoperative physician's and anesthetist's opinion should be obtained. Diabetes and hypertension should be well controlled. Anemia should be corrected.
- Skeletal and neuromuscular deformities making lithotomy position difficult, should be taken into consideration.

POINTS IN CLINICAL EXAMINATIONS THAT ARE IMPORTANT FOR CASE SELECTION (TABLE 1)

See **Table 1**

IMPORTANT FACTORS INFLUENCING THE DECISION OF VAGINAL HYSTERECTOMY (TABLE 2)

See **Table 2**

TABLE 1: Clinical examinations which are important for case selection.

P/A examination	*P/S examination*	*P/V examination*	*P/R examination*	*USG*
• Size and shape of uterus if palpable • If large, then mobility • Quality and number of scars of previous surgeries • Lifting anterior abdominal wall to assess fixity and adhesions • Lump—uterine or ovarian mass, differentiated clinically	• Position of cervix, approachability from vaginal route with and without traction with vulsellum and on coughing also • Cystocele, Rectocele, Enterocele, Urethrocele, Pelvic organ prolapse, Complete procidentia • Descent of cervix, urinary incontinence, bulging in area of enterocele on coughing • Invisible or barely visible cervix • Very short / hypertrophied/torn/Ulcerated cervix • Narrow vagina, cicatrization, fibrosis due to birth trauma, post- menopausal atrophic changes, shallow or obliterated fornices	• Size and shape of uterus • Mobility and assessment • Adhesions with anterior abdominal wall and previous scars • Consistency of tissue • Obliterated fornices, cul-de-sac assessment, if obliterated then its proximity to rectum • Assessment of adnexal mass, size and cause	• Possibility of rectosigmoid endometriosis should be considered	• Size, shape, volume and weight of uterus • Number, size, location and vascularity of fibroids, mapping of fibroids • Adnexal mass—ovarian pathology, approachability from vaginal route

TABLE 2: Factor for deciding the vaginal hysterectomy.

	Factors to be considered	*Average case*	*Difficult case—need for concurrent procedures*	*Remarks*
1	Size of uterus, assessed by clinical examination and USG	• Up to 12 weeks • Can be easily removed	12–22 weeks will require: • Morcellation • Bisection • Coring • Enucleation of fibroids by myoma screw • Lateral cut leaving large area of TO • Pedicle which will be dealt afterwards	Depends up on experience, skill, modification in technique and confidence of surgeon
2	• Shape of uterus and deviation—assessed by clinical examination and USG • Fibroids or adhesions or adnexal mass	• Preoperative assessment is very useful • Uterus should be palpated separate from mass	• Remain close to uterus • Sharp dissection in proper plane	• Gradual traction on cervix will help in achieving descent • It will also decrease blood loss by narrowing lumen of blood vessels
3	• Adhesions due to previous surgeries—cesarean section, hysterotomy, sterilization, ectopic pregnancy • Pelvic inflammatory disease or endometriosis or bowel disease or adnexal pathology	• Adhesions with urinary bladder are easily excised with sharp dissection • Irrespective of number of scars. • Adhesion of uterus with anterior abdominal wall will require help of laparoscopy. Pouches will open on their own during surgery. An unnecessary attempt to open pouches may lead to inadvertent injury	• Perfect planning • Use of energy sources	With increasing experience and better technique, more and more difficult cases will be operated easily

Contd...

Contd...

	Factors to be considered	*Average case*	*Difficult case—need for concurrent procedures*	*Remarks*
4	Space in vagina, accessibility of cervix, short cervix, shallow or obliterated fornices, fibrosis, torn cervix, injury to cervix while catching with vulsellum, limited lateral space, tough tissue especially very strong uterosacral ligaments, hypertrophied large cervix	• Descent is achieved once uterosacral and cardinal ligaments are clamped, cut and ligated or excised with sealer • Limited lateral space is not a problem with use of energy sources	Experience of working in narrow space with minimal instruments in the surgical field is helpful	
5	• Training, skill, expertise and experience of surgeon and assistants • Available technology in hospital for limb support, position and devices like vessel sealer	• Easy to learn from an experienced surgeon under his supervision • Straight leg raising position has distinct advantages		• Good technique • Day-to-day learning • Improvement with open mind • Use of energy sources • Gradually more and more difficult cases will be managed

ABSOLUTE CONTRAINDICATIONS OF VAGINAL HYSTERECTOMY

- Large uterus more than 22 weeks size
- Multiple large fibroids, not approachable vaginally including broad ligament fibroid
- Large tubo-ovarian mass inseparable from uterus
- Obliterated cul de sac due to dense adhesions of rectosigmoid and rectovaginal endometriosis
- Multiple scars with dense bowel and omental adhesions of uterus with anterior abdominal wall.
  Fundus and posterior surface of uterus inseparable from adhesions.
- Invisible short cervix, pulled upwards not approachable
- Advanced malignancy of cervix, uterus and ovaries
- Mullerian anomalies affecting vagina.

Ideally all uteri should be removed vaginally if possible. Laparoscopic hysterectomy is a preferred alternative to abdominal hysterectomy and in cases when vaginal hysterectomy is not indicated or not feasible. Laparoscopic hysterectomy has limitations like higher cost, expensive instruments, longer learning curve and morbidity depending upon surgeon's expertise.[3]

Vaginal hysterectomy is a better option than abdominal hysterectomy as it is feasible, safe and provides more patient comfort without increasing duration of surgery, intraoperative and postoperative complications.[4]

This minimal access surgery is no hole surgery through natural orifice, studies have shown that vaginal hysterectomy is the most beneficial method compared to other methods, and it is associated with least complications.[5]

For a case of pelvic organ prolapse, the decision to preserve/remove uterus along with repair of the defect is important. Failure to detect defects followed by hysterectomy without proper repair will end up in vault prolapse or a large cystocele and/rectocele or urinary incontinence later.

CONCLUSION

Vaginal hysterectomy is possible in 85–90% of cases. Only 10–15% will require total laparoscopic hysterectomy/laparoscopic assistance or abdominal hysterectomy. Selection of patients for vaginal hysterectomy is the crucial decision which depends on history, thorough clinical examination and skill of surgeon. Perfect clinical judgement of operating surgeons, advance planning for help from laparoscopic intervention, assessment of difficulties and management plan to overcome them during surgery and skill and confidence of surgeon are essential factors for successful VH.

REFERENCES

1. Committee Opinion No 701: Choosing the route of hysterectomy for benign disease. Obstet Gynecol. 2017;129(6):e155-9. doi: 10.1097/AOG.0000000000002112. PMID: 28538495.
2. The Journal of Obstetrics and Gynecology of India (July-August 2015) 65(4):251-4. DOI 10.1007/s13224- 014-0562-z.
3. The Journal of Obstetrics and Gynecology of India (January-February 2015) 65(1):39-44. DOI 10.1007/s 13224-014-0578-4.
4. MedPulse—International Journal of Gynecology, IISN: 2579-0870, Online ISSN: 2636-4719, Volume 12, Issue 3, December 2019.
5. Gupta M, Jindal M, Goraya SPS. A Study on deciding the route of hysterectomy. Int Arch BioMed Clin Res. 2017;3(3):42-4. DOI:10.21276/iabcr.2017.3.3.11.

3 CHAPTER

Patient Positioning in Vaginal Surgeries

Rajeshree Jain

INTRODUCTION

Positioning of patients is vital for dynamics and ergonomics of vaginal surgeries.

There are small yet very important points to be considered and incorporated into reflexes for comfortable and safe surgery. Ideally, there is significant preoperative assessment for positioning as well.

PREOPERATIVE ASSESSMENT

1. Age/height/weight/BMI.
2. Internal/external devices, prosthesis and implants.
3. Previous surgeries, like total knee replacement, hip or spine surgery.
4. Preexisting conditions:
   i. Osteoarthritis, especially hip and knee joints, limiting the hip and knee mobility.
   ii. Better simulate the position in preoperative awake and aware patient, to look for unequal mobility and asymmetry.
   iii. Lumbar disc prolapse may get exacerbated.
   iv. Osteoporosis which may lead to fracture and dislocation.
   v. Varicosities, risk of deep vein thrombosis.
   vi. Skin integrity especially, for cautery plate and pressure points.
   vii. Medical history and investigations for comorbidities of CVS, RS and DM as diabetic neuropathies are common.

In head-down Trendelenburg position by 15°, diaphragm is pushed up which compromises with respiration especially in obese patients. It facilitates increased venous return, and increased cardiac output, especially in hypertensive patients **(Fig. 1)**.

SETTING LITHOTOMY POSITION

- Buttocks should be just at the edge of the table in supine position.
- With legs separated and flexed at hip and knee joints.

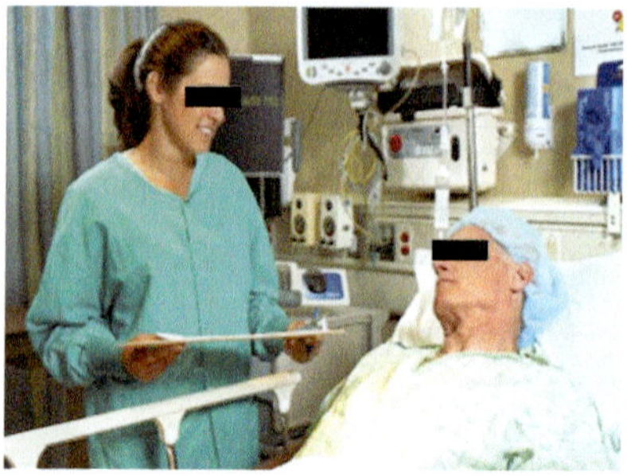

Fig. 1: History taking and preoperative assessment.

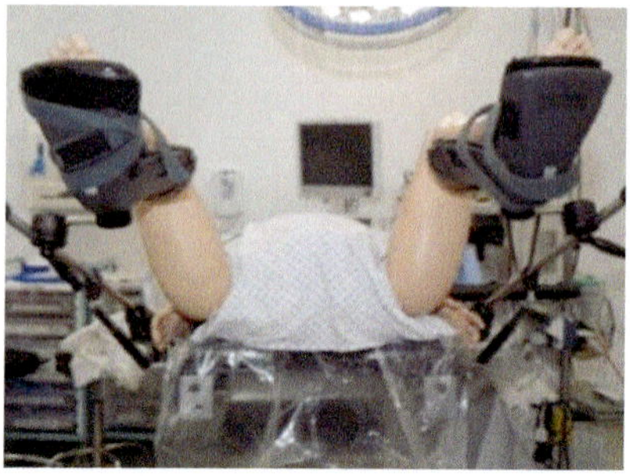

Fig. 2: Lithotomy position for vaginal surgeries.

- Preferably hips 80–100° from trunk, with slight abduction 30–45° from midline **(Fig. 2)**.
- Legs supported in raised stirrups **(Figs. 3 to 5)**.

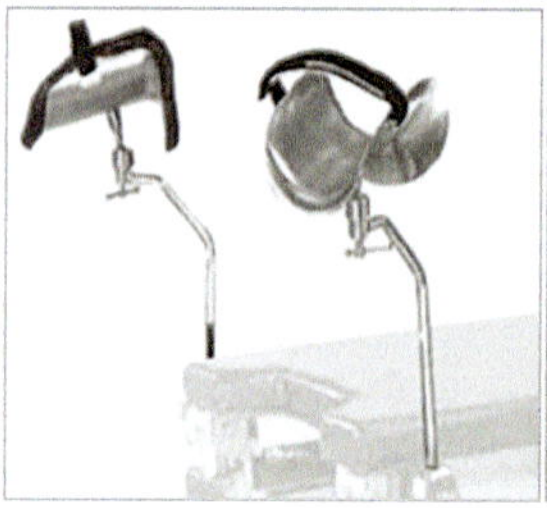

Fig. 3: Knee crutch.

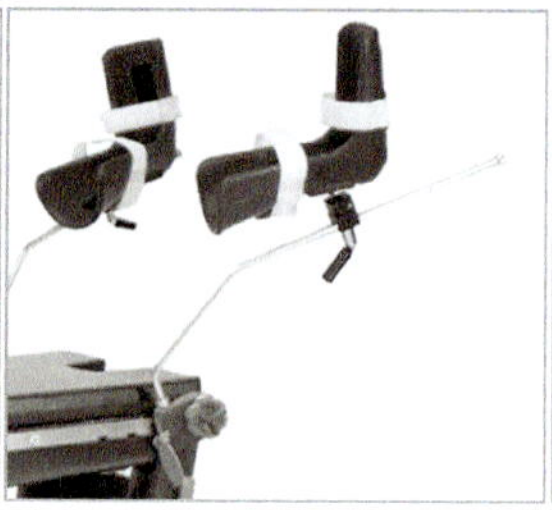

Fig. 4: Boot support.

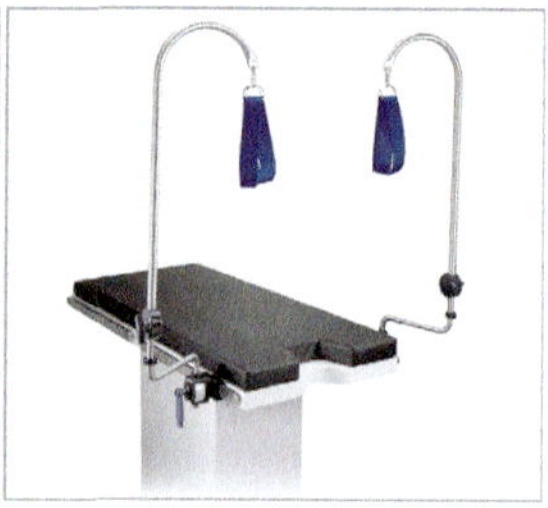

Fig. 5: Candy cane.

Precaution is taken to elevate both the legs simultaneously by two OT staff, to avoid strain at hip and SI joints. Pressure points should be nicely padded, and straps should not be tightened at nerve locations.

Height of table, and height of surgeon's stool should be adjusted, so that operating field should be in line with surgeon's eye and two assistants should stand within the stirrup, one on either side.

Preferable to keep instruments tray on surgeon's lap **(Fig. 6)**.

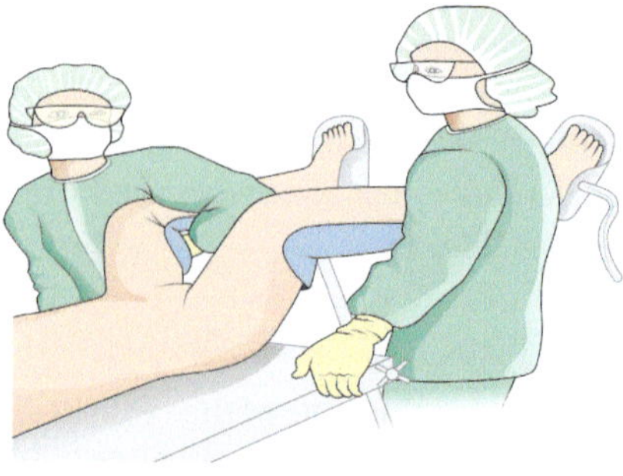

Fig. 6: Elevate both legs simultaneously.

UPPER LIMB CARE

Be careful about supporting the upper limb. They should be supported on arm rest, making less than 90° angle at axilla because extension of arm above 90° for long time, causes traction of brachial plexus. Watch patients hands to avoid crush injury while repositing table back **(Fig. 7)**.

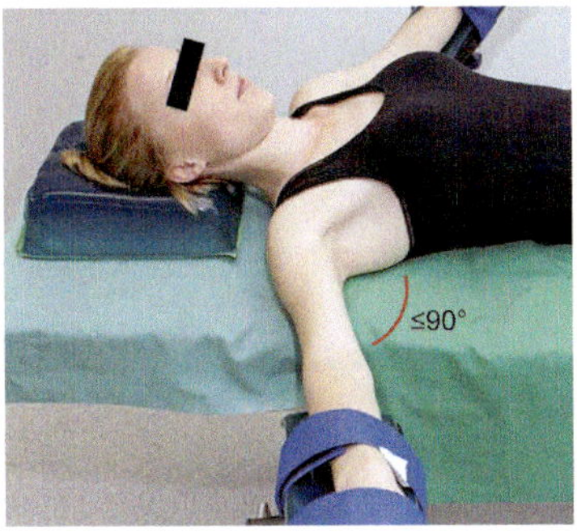

Fig. 7: Upper limb care.

OBESE PATIENT

Modified lithotomy position is adapted for obese and super-obese patients for surgeons' comfort and safety of patient in order to **(Fig. 8)**:

- Avoid pressure points and give extra paddings
- Ease joints and ligaments
- Retract extra soft tissues with taping
- Overhead light
- DVT precautions (DVT pumps)
- Considerations for cardiopulmonary extra care
- Prolonged positioning to be kept in mind
- Special OT table required

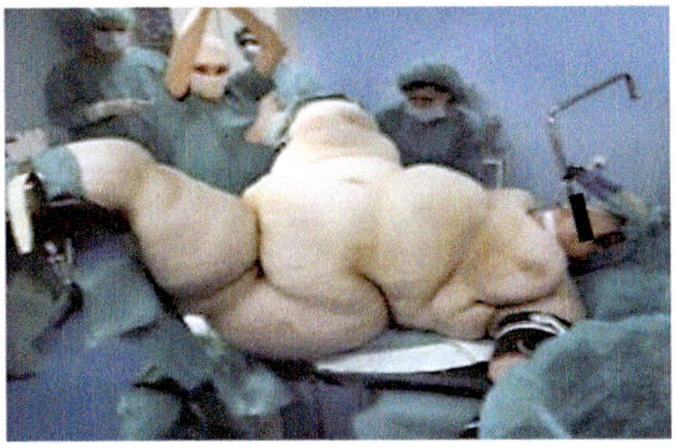

Fig. 8: Modified lithotomy in obese patients.

ENERGY SOURCE

Avoid body contact with metal surfaces to avoid earthing and electric injuries or burns. Ornaments to be removed or insulated. The cautery plate/pad should be in a good large area of contact avoiding joints, bony contours and superficial nerves. Pacemakers and Implants are taken into account while placing of cautery grounding plate/pad avoiding circuit interference.

SHIFTING OF PATIENT

Lifting the patient on stretch-out sheath from shoulder to pelvic girdle, from OT table to trolley with head neck and legs supported. Because lifting on folded sheath at lumber curve, can cause hyper extension injury of lumbar spine **(Figs. 9 and 10)**.

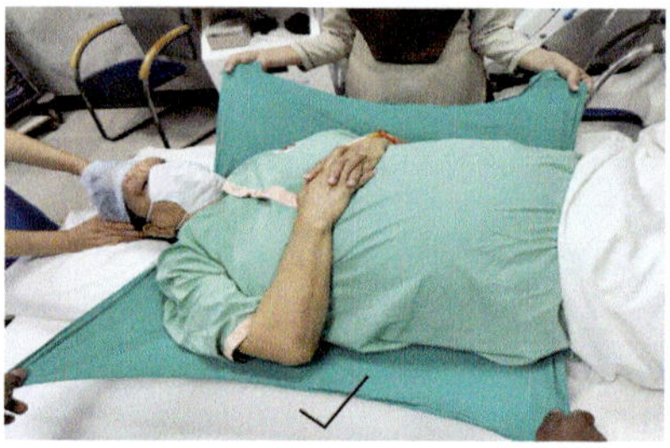

Fig. 9: The right way of lifting patient.

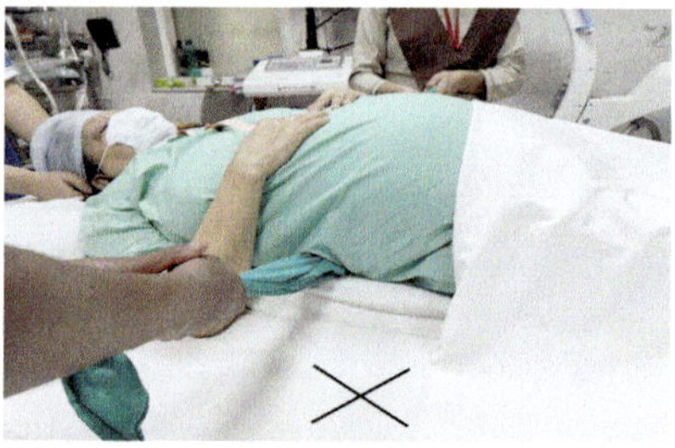

Fig. 10: Wrong way of lifting patient.

NEUROPRAXIA

Focal blocking of impulse conduction is limited to affected nerve segments. May be attributed to brief interruption of blood supply due to external compression, where recovery can take hours, days, weeks, or months depending upon initial insult. It exhibits as reduced sensory perception and/or motor weakness in extremities with diffuse pain.

LITHOTOMY: NEURALGIAS OF CONCERN

Peroneal and Saphenous Nerve Insult

Most common nerve compression insult is to common peroneal nerve at neck of fibula by bar or supports for which padding with cotton or foam is preferable. Also seen is saphenous nerve insult due to pressure at tibial condyle and ankle **(Figs. 11 to 13)**.

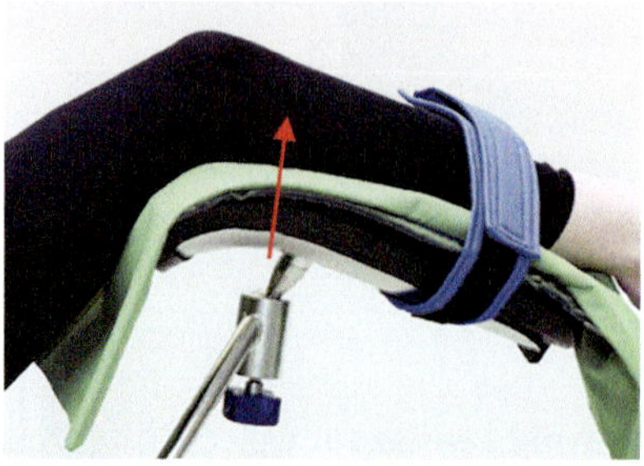

Fig. 11: Strap away from common peroneal nerve (arrow).

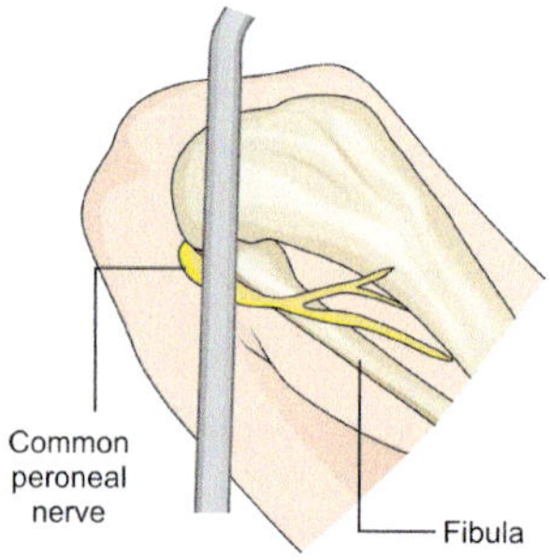

Fig. 12: Common peroneal nerve compression by bar.

HYPERFLEXION OF HIP

- Causes stretching of sciatic nerve, obturator nerve as it exits obturator foramen.
- Increased lumbar intradiscal pressure especially in preexisting lumbar disc disease.

PROLONG GROIN FOLDING

- Causes bending of femoral nerve and pressing against inguinal ligament.
- Postoperative deficits in hip flexion and knee extension with reduced patellar reflex.
- Compression on lateral cutaneous nerve of thigh leading to tingling and numbness in anterolateral thigh, meralgia paresthetica. Possibility of vascular compression and compromise should be kept in mind **(Fig. 14)**.

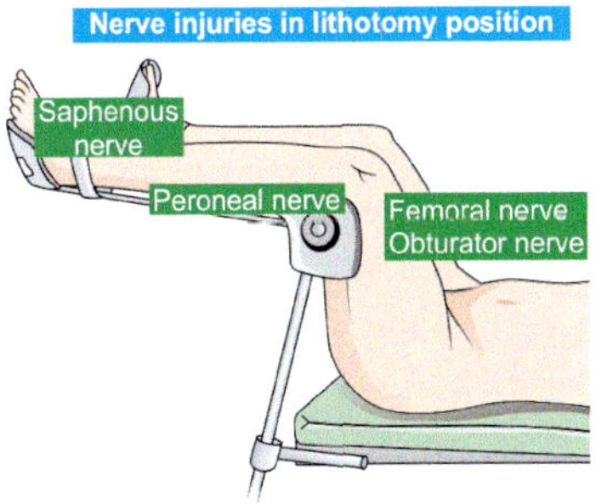

Fig. 13: Peroneal, saphenous, femoral, and obturator nerves.

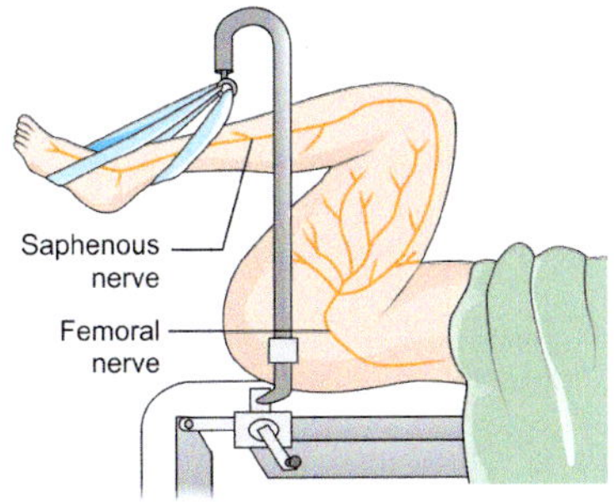

Fig. 14: Prolonged groin-folding femoral nerve insult.

HYPERABDUCTION OF THIGH WITH EXTERNAL ROTATION

Risking hip dislocation, fracture in severely osteoporotic patients. Implants and prosthesis need special considerations.

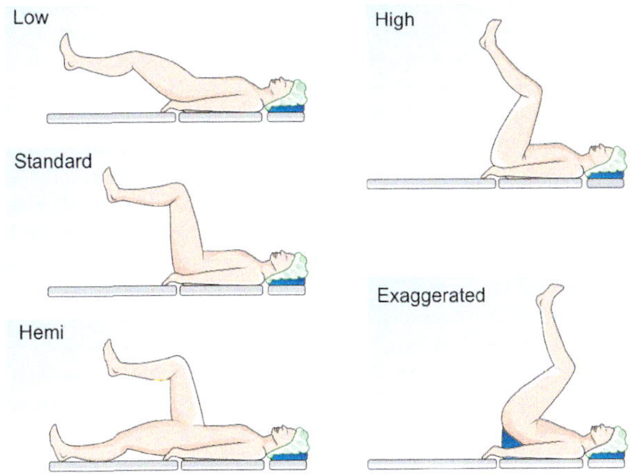

Lithotomy—adjusted

CONCLUSION

Positioning of patients is important for good surgical access with maximum comfort to surgeon and assisting team and to avoid risk or complications including:

Hemodynamic instability
- Impaired ventilation
- Neuropraxia
- Musculoskeletal injury
- Exacerbation of disc problems
- Cautery burn injury
- Venous thrombosis
- Compartment syndrome (very rare)

May be AI in future may guide us for customized position, according to pooled patients' data.

Till then introspect about proper positioning. So always be cautious and conscious about positioning.

SUGGESTED READING

1. Bauer ECA, Koch N, Erichsen CJ. Survey of compartment syndrome of the lower extremity after gynecological operations. Langenbeck's Arch Surg. 2014;399:343-8.
2. DOI http://dx.doi.org/10.1055/s-0035-1557776 Geburtsh Frauenheilk 2015; 75: 792–807 © Georg Thieme Verlag KG Stuttgart. New York. ISSN 0016-5751.
3. Karmaniolou I, Staikou C. Compartment syndrome as a complication of the lithotomy position. West Indian Med J. 2010;59(6):698-701.
4. Kuponiyi O, Alleemudder D, Latunde-Dada A, Eedarapalli P. Nerve injuries associated with gynaecological surgery. Obstet Gynaecol. 2014;16(1):29-36.
5. Litwiller JP, Wells RE, Halliwill JR. Effect of lithotomy positions on strain of the obturator and lateral femoral cutaneous nerves. Clin Anat. 2004;17:45-9.
6. Recommendations for Preventing Positioning-Related Damage in Surgical Gynecology. Guideline of the DGGG, OEGGG and SGGG. Obstetrics and Gynaecology 2021;81(4):447-8.
7. Warner MA, Warner DO, Harper CM. Lower extremity neuropathies associated with lithotomy positions. Anesthesiology. 2000;93:938-42.

4

CHAPTER

Comprehensive Clinical Evaluation and Assessment of Pelvic Organ Prolapse

Richa Narkhade

INTRODUCTION

Pelvic organ prolapse (POP) is a significant yet frequently overlooked gynecological condition, affecting millions of women worldwide particularly among women in Asia. Many individuals tend to dismiss early symptoms, often leading to worsening conditions that adversely affect quality of life.[1] Despite its prevalence, this condition remains underreported and under-recognized, especially among Asian women. Cultural stigmas, lack of awareness, and limited access to healthcare contribute to the neglect of early symptoms, which can lead to severe physical and psychological consequences. Therefore, it is essential to provide thorough knowledge about POP to empower patients in recognizing symptoms early and seeking appropriate care. Pelvic organ prolapse (POP) refers to the descent of pelvic structures into the vagina, resulting from weakness in the ligaments or muscles that support these organs **(Table 1)**.

Pelvic organ prolapse (POP) may affect one or more of the vaginal compartments, which are categorized as follows:[2]

CENTRAL AND LATERAL CYSTOCELE

Central defects arise from vertical weaknesses in the endopelvic fascia, while lateral defects result from the detachment of the lateral vaginal wall from the arcus tendineus fascia pelvis. Central defects are further categorized into anterior and posterior types. Prolapse occurring anterior to the interureteric bar (also known as Mercier's bar) is referred to as an anterior cystocele or urethrovaginal prolapse. Conversely, prolapse posterior to Mercier's bar is classified as a posterior cystocele.[3]

These conditions can present individually or in combination. While the causes of POP are multifaceted, there is a significant correlation with pregnancy and vaginal delivery, which can cause direct injury to the pelvic floor muscles and connective tissues.

TABLE 1: Anatomical classification according to vaginal walls (enterocele can also be seen in the posterior compartment).

Anterior vaginal wall (Anterior compartment)	*Cystocele:* • Central (Posterior) • Lateral (Anterior) • Combined	*Urethrocele:* Uncommon
Apical vaginal wall (Middle compartment)	*Enterocele uterine:* • Anterior • Posterior	*Uterovaginal; vaginal vault:* With cystocele, enterocele, rectocele; eversion (post-hysterectomy) with cystocele, enterocele, rectocele
Posterior vaginal wall (Posterior compartment)	*Rectocele:* • Low • Midvaginal	

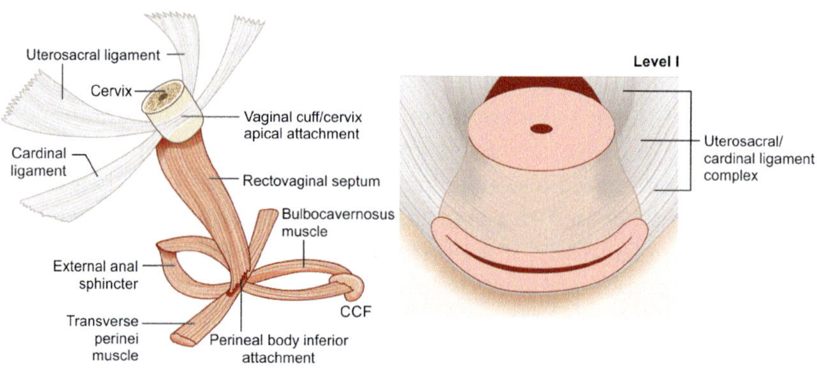

Fig. 1: *Level I:* The cardinal uterosacral ligament complex.

Classification of Pelvic Organ Prolapse

Pelvic organ support is maintained by complex interactions between the vagina, levator ani muscle, and pelvic floor connective tissue. A system of three integrated levels of vaginal support has been described by De Lancey **(Figs. 1 to 3)**.

CLINICAL ASSESSMENT

Patient History

Symptom Inquiry

Begin with a detailed assessment of symptoms. Common complaints include:

- *Pelvic pressure:* A feeling of heaviness or fullness in the pelvic area.
- *Bulging:* Sensation or visibility of a bulge in the vagina or perineum.
- *Urinary symptoms:* Incontinence, urgency, frequency, or incomplete bladder emptying.

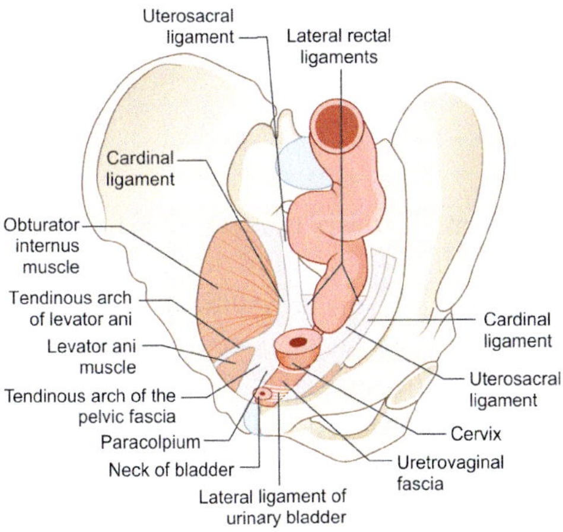

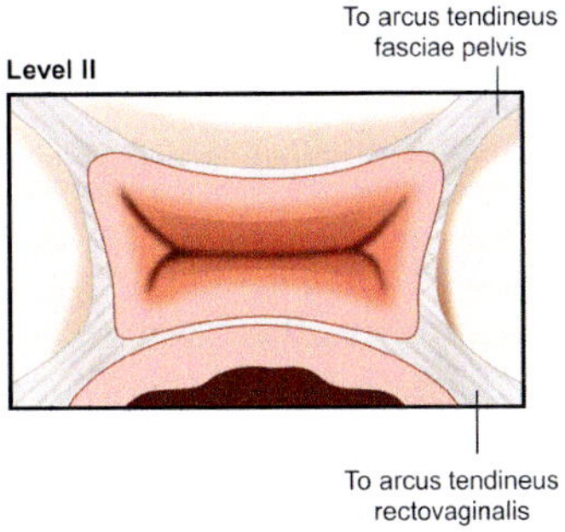

Fig. 2: *Level II* support comprises the paravaginal attachments that run the length of the vagina and are suspended by the arcus tendineus fasciae pelvis (ATFP), or lateral pelvic white line. Loss of level II support contributes to cystocele (anterior vaginal prolapse)

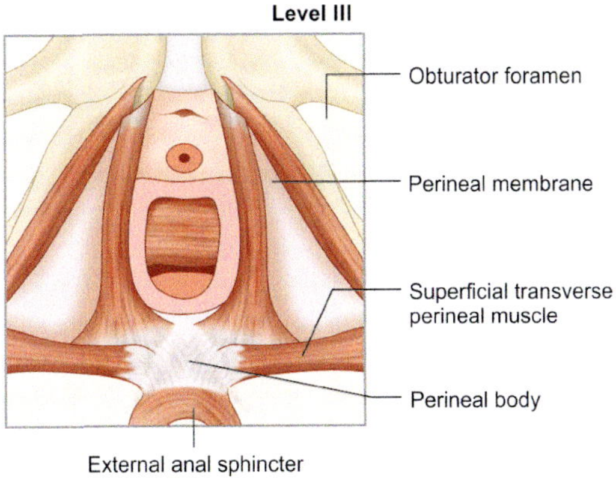

Fig. 3: *Level III:* Urogenital diaphragm and the perineal body.

- *Bowel symptoms:* Constipation, fecal incontinence, or a feeling of incomplete evacuation.
- *Sexual dysfunction (with permission):* Pain during intercourse or changes in sexual desire.

Obstetric and Gynecological History

Document relevant details, including:

- Number of pregnancies and deliveries (both vaginal—instrumental and cesarean)
- Any history of pelvic or abdominal surgeries
- Menstrual history and any history of gynecological disorders

- *Medical history:* Chronic conditions such as obesity, chronic cough, and connective tissue disorders (e.g., Ehlers-Danlos syndrome) can contribute to prolapse.

Physical Examination

The examination commences as soon as the patient enters the room. Observing her appearance and gait can offer valuable insights into how prolapse impacts her quality of life. A comprehensive examination is crucial for identifying the presence and extent of prolapse. Key steps include:[4]

1. Before initiating the examination, ensure the patient has a full bladder. Provide privacy and instruct her to stand and spread her legs. Ask her to perform a Valsalva maneuver or cough to help identify any instances of stress incontinence.
2. *Positioning:* Evaluate the patient in both supine and standing positions to effectively assess the extent of prolapse. Encourage her to cough during these assessments to further evaluate any changes.
3. *Visual inspection:* Look for signs of prolapse, including the degree of descent, keratinization, decubitus ulcers, and edema **(Fig. 4)**.

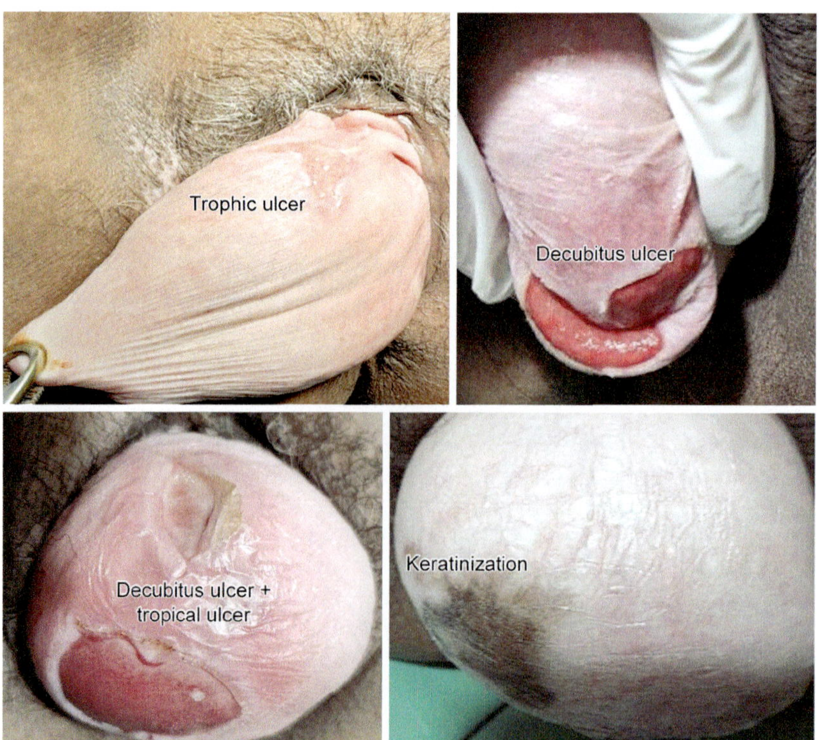

Fig. 4: Visual inspection.

4. *Speculum examination:* Identify cervical elongation under traction, noting any compartment defects and assessing perineal laxity **(Fig. 5)**.

Pop-Q System

Employ the Pelvic Organ Prolapse Quantification (POP-Q) system for standardized measurement of prolapse **(Table 2)**. The International Continence Society (ICS) has adopted the POP-Q system in 1996 introduced by Dr Richard Bump and further approved by the American Urogynecologic Society (AUGS), Society of Gynecologic Surgeons (SGS), and recently by National Institute of Health (NIH).[3,5]

- *Measurements:* Based on anatomical landmarks, particularly the hymen. The POP-Q system provides a detailed framework for assessing the topographic positions of six vaginal sites.[5,6] It evaluates perineal descent and the changes in the axis of the levator plate. This assessment is based

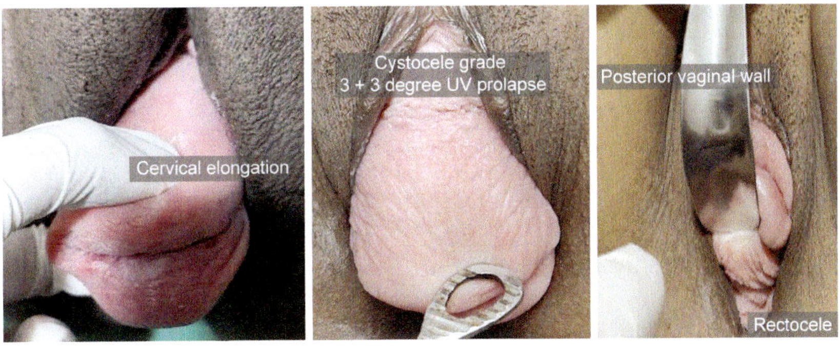

Fig. 5: Speculum examination.

TABLE 2: Staging of pelvic organ prolapse according to pelvic organ prolapse quantification (POP-Q) system.

Stage of prolapse	Extent of prolapse (in relationship to the hymen: prolapse above the hymen, negative numbers; prolapse beyond the hymen, positive numbers)
Stage 0	No prolapse (apex can descend as far as 2 cm relative to the total vaginal length)
Stage I	The most portion of prolapse descends to a point less more than 1 cm above the hymen
Stage II	Maximum descent is within 1 cm of the hymen
Stage III	Prolapse extends more than 1 cm beyond the hymen but no more than 2 cm of the total vaginal length
Stage IV	Complete eversion of the vagina or descent within 2 cm of the total vaginal length

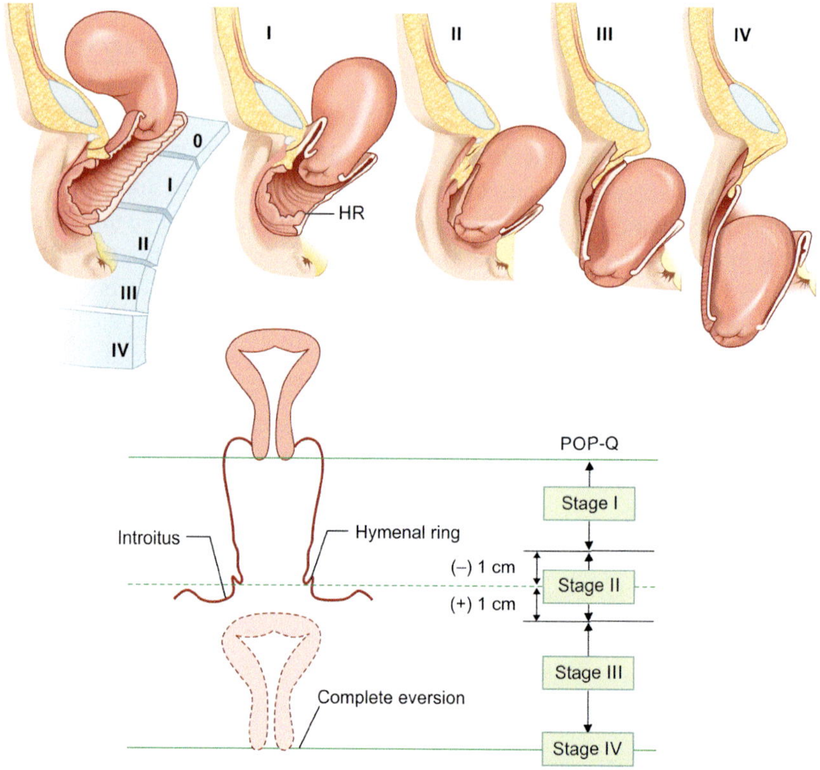

Fig. 6: The POP-Q system provides a detailed framework for assessing the topographic positions of six vaginal sites.

on precise measurements of the genital hiatus and perineal body, allowing for a thorough understanding of pelvic organ support and the degree of prolapse, the middle quadrant consists of the genital hiatus, perineal body, and total vaginal length, measured after complete repositioning of the prolapse, followed by the other six measurements during maximum Valsalva **(Fig. 6)**.[7]

- *Classification:* Prolapse severity is categorized into stages ranging from 0 to IV **(Fig. 7)**.[8]

Assessment of Symptoms

Utilize validated questionnaires to quantify the impact of pelvic symptoms on quality of life. Common tools include:

- *Pelvic floor distress inventory (PFDI):* Assesses distress from pelvic floor disorders.
- *Pelvic floor impact questionnaire (PFIQ):* Evaluates the impact on daily activities and quality of life.

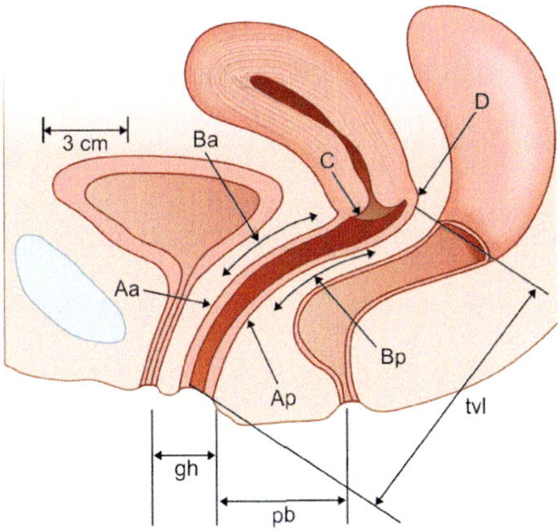

Anterior wall Aa	Anterior wall Ba	Cervix or cuff C
Genital hiatus gH	Perineal body pB	Total vaginal length TVL
Posterior wall Ap	Posterior wall Bp	Posterior fornix D

Fig. 7: POP-Q points. Aa, anterior vaginal wall 3 cm proximal to the urethral meatus (–3 cm to +3 cm); Ba, most distal position of the remaining upper anterior vaginal wall (–3 cm to +tvl); C, most distal edge of cervix or vaginal cuff scar; D, posterior fornix (n/a if posthysterectomy); Ap, posterior vaginal wall 3 cm proximal to the hymen (–3 cm to +3 cm); Bp, most distal position of the remaining upper posterior vaginal wall (–3 cm to +tvl); genital hiatus (gh), measured from the middle of external urethral meatus to the posterior midline hymen; perineal body (pb), measured from the posterior margin of gh to the middle of anal opening; total vaginal length (tvl), depth of the vagina when point D or C is reduced to normal position.[9]

Diagnostic Tools

Imaging Studies

- *Ultrasound:* Transvaginal or abdominal ultrasound can help visualize pelvic organ anatomy, assess the presence of prolapse, and identify any structural abnormalities.
- *MRI:* Magnetic resonance imaging provides detailed images of pelvic structures and can be particularly useful in complex cases or when planning surgical intervention.

Urodynamic Studies

These studies assess bladder function and can help differentiate between urinary incontinence due to prolapse and other underlying urological conditions. Tests may include:

- *Uroflowmetry:* Measures the flow rate of urine.
- *Cytometry:* Evaluates bladder capacity and pressure during filling.
- *Pressure flow studies:* Assesses bladder pressure during voiding.

Defecography

For patients presenting with bowel symptoms, defecography evaluates the mechanics of defecation and can identify conditions such as rectocele or other structural issues affecting bowel function.

CONCLUSION

The evaluation of pelvic organ prolapse requires a thorough assessment that encompasses clinical history, physical examination, and diagnostic tools. Understanding the severity and impact of symptoms is crucial for effective management. Both conservative and surgical options should be considered based on individual patient circumstances, with the goal of improving quality of life and functional outcomes.

REFERENCES

1. Jokhio AH, Rizvi RM, MacArthur C. Prevalence of pelvic organ prolapse in women, associated factors and impact on quality of life in rural Pakistan: population-based study. BMC Womens Health. 2020;20(1):82. doi: 10.1186/s12905-020-00934-6. PMID: 32345271; PMCID: PMC7189438.
2. Persu C, Chapple CR, Cauni V, Gutue S, Geavlete P. Pelvic organ prolapse quantification system (POP-Q): a new era in pelvic prolapse staging. J Med Life. 2011;4(1):75-81. Epub 2011 Feb 25. PMID: 21505577; PMCID: PMC3056425.
3. Gharib EL. Central and lateral cystocele. Sci J Research & Rev. 2018;1(1):ID.000505. DOI: 10.33552/SJRR.2018.01.000505.
4. Bhadana P. Pelvic organ prolapse: examination and assessment [Internet]. Lower urinary tract dysfunction—from evidence to clinical practice. IntechOpen; 2020. Available from: http://dx.doi.org/10.5772/intechopen.91357.
5. Digesu GA, Athanasiou S, Cardozo L, et al. Validation of the pelvic organ prolapse quantification (POP-Q) system in left lateral position. Int Urogynecological J. 2009;20(8):979-83. DOI: 10.1007/s00192-009-0884-z.
6. Kobak WH, Rosenberger K, Walters MD. Interobserver variation in the assessment of pelvic organ prolapse. Int Urogynecol J. 1996;7(3):121-4. DOI: 10.1007/BF01894199.
7. Raizada N, Mittal P, Suri J, et al. Comparative study to evaluate the intersystem association and reliability between standard pelvic organ prolapse quantification system and simplified pelvic organ prolapse scoring system. J Obstet Gynecol India. 2014;64(6):421-4. DOI: 10.1007/s13224-014-0537-0.
8. Muta, N. Pelvic floor muscle training for pelvic organ prolapse: pelvic floor rehabilitation in our hospital. Japanese Journal of Physical Fitness and Sports Medicine. 2022;71:263-9. 10.7600/jspfsm.71.263.
9. Duddalwar VA, Bhalerao A. Comparative Study to Evaluate Intersystem Association between Pelvic Organ Prolapse Quantification System and Simplified Pelvic Organ Prolapse Scoring System. J South Asian Feder Obst Gynae 2021;13(5):325-9.

5 CHAPTER

OT Set Up and Instrumentation for Vaginal Surgery

Ashok Kumar Todani, Kiran Lata Todani

Effective and successful surgery is not only dependent on the surgeon's judgment and technical competence, but also on the choice of appropriately designed operation theater, designed instruments, trained staff and superb postoperative care.

In obstetrics, episiotomy is the most common vaginal operation performed in day-to-day practice. After cesarean section, hysterectomy is the most common surgery in gynecologic practice.

An operating theater [also known as an operating room (OR), operating suite, or operation suite] is a facility within a hospital, where surgical operations are carried out in an aseptic environment.

Why You Might Need Vaginal Surgery?

Any woman whose urovaginal region has been altered or injured for various medical reasons may be eligible for vaginal surgical intervention and plasty. Among the many candidates for reconstructive procedures are:

- Cancer patients who underwent extensive surgery or radiation treatments for cancer of the organs and structures of the urinary tract and/or reproductive system.
- Women with uterine/vaginal wall prolapse, uterine neoplasia.
- Women who have physical trauma to the vaginal region as a result of accident, childbirth, assault, or rape.
- Women with congenital abnormalities (birth defects) affecting the vaginal region.

OPERATION THEATER

Basic Set-up of OT (OR)

- The operating theater should be accommodating to safe surgery and anesthesia and should be at least 7 × 7 meters with a ceiling height of 3.5 meters.
- Separated from the main flow of hospital traffic
- It should be easily accessible from surgical wards and emergency rooms.

- The floor should be covered with antistatic material.
- The walls should be painted with impervious, antistatic paint (reduces the dust levels and allows frequent cleaning).
- The surfaces must withstand frequent cleaning and decontamination with disinfectant.

Layout of Operating Theater (Figs. 1 and 2)

- Clean corridor scrub-up area
- Recovery area
- Anesthetic room sterile supplies store

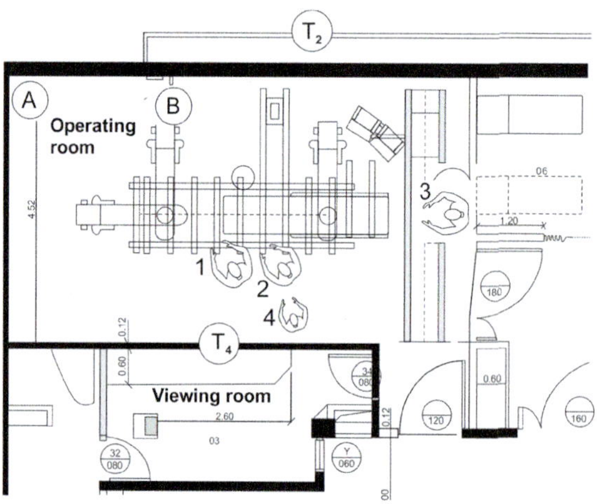

Fig. 1: Layout of operation theater.

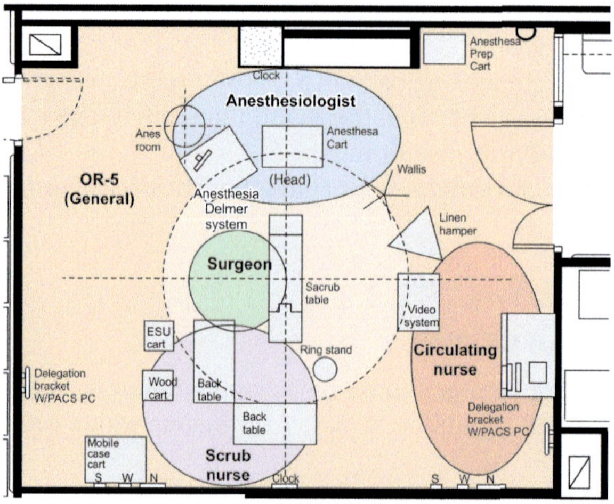

Fig. 2: Operating room work zones.

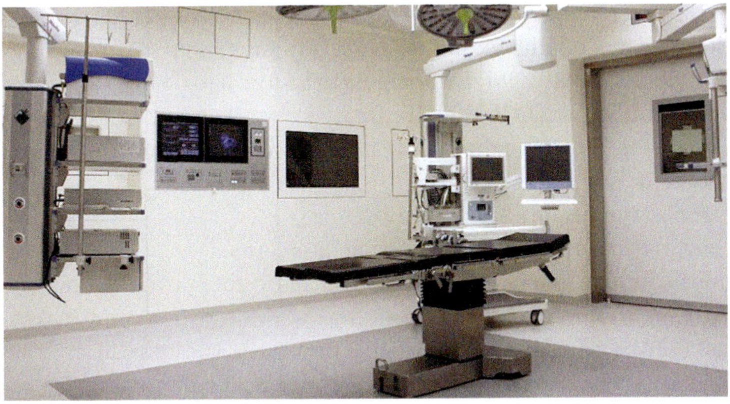

Fig. 3: Modular operation theater for hospital operating room.

Types of OT/OR

- *Hybrid OR:* Hybrid operating room requirements are usually based around imaging, like CT, MR, C-arm or other types of imaging, being brought into surgery.
- *Integrated OR:* As video routing systems capable of distributing video signals from one camera to multiple outputs or products. Patient information, audio, video, surgical and room lights, building automation, and specialized equipment, including imaging devices, could all communicate with one another.
- *Digital OR:* A digital OR is a setup in which software sources, images and operating room video integration is made possible.

Modular OT/OR

Modular OT: It is the ultramodern and ultraclean OT matching all international sterility protocols and standards **(Fig. 3)**.

Modular OT Specifications

- *Absolute flatness*
- *Vertical level adjustment of subframe*
- *Hermetic sealing*
- *Sound insulation*
- *Non-flammable materials*
- *Ease of disassembly—individuality of panels*

How to Prepare for Vaginal Surgery?

While every woman is different and the various purposes for these procedures are varied, the intended result of these surgeries are similar:

- Facilitate childbirth
- Correction of pathology and relief of symptoms
- In vaginoplasty, to tighten the vagina to restore it to nearly the same size it was before experiencing childbirth.
- Improving the appearance of the labia can lead to a boost in self-confidence.
- Exercise can become more comfortable.
- Heightened sensitivity during sexual intercourse
- Improvements in self-perception and self-esteem can enhance quality of life.

It should be noted that while it is true that vaginal tissues can stretch, such as what is experienced during childbirth, surgically tightening the vaginal tissue on its own does not guarantee a heightened sexual response. In fact, heightened sexual sensitivity is not an automatic guarantee for more pleasure and can instead lead to oversensitivity and pain.

Preparation for surgery depends on the type of surgery being performed and what the needs of the reconstruction or rejuvenation are. Your doctor will offer several recommendations that you will need to follow prior to your surgical procedure and are common to most surgeries.

Additionally, vaginal reconstruction or rejuvenation is a great option for a woman in good health who has one or more of the following concerns:

- The contours of the genital structures have become inelastic or stretched out
- Soreness or pain with sexual activity or exercise
- Diminished sensation during intercourse proceeding childbirth
- A desire to improve the contour or appearance of the genitals

Vaginal reconstruction or vaginal rejuvenation surgery are the terms used for a wide range of procedures whose objectives are to repair or reconstruct the vagina. Vaginal surgery of this kind aims to reduce pain and improve the appearance, size, function and possibly the sensitivity of the vagina.

BASIC REQUIREMENTS

Anesthesia Machine and Life-saving Accessories

Anesthesia machine having latest gadgets including induction, maintenance, resuscitation, defibrillator and all other accessories to tackle any emergency are a must.

Lighting: Be adequate to illuminate operating field efficiently. When this is directed over the right-handed surgeon's left shoulder, illumination should be shadow-free. LED light sources are used these days. Wearing a fiberoptic or tungsten headlight, which will provide a shadowless spot from 2 to 4 inches of very bright light in the center of the operative field.

Operating table: The operating table to be used for vaginal surgery should be equipped with adjustable stirrups that can be extended at least 15 inches or more suitable to leg length of patient. When a patient's ankles are suspended from the stirrups, acute angulation of the leg will be avoided to ensure unobstructed venous return. The operating table should be equipped to ensure rapid adjustment into the varying degrees of Trendelenburg and reverse Trendelenburg positions as per need. Elastic stockings for the patient are advisable and should be in place before induction of anesthesia to avoid venous thrombosis.

Manual or motorized operating tables may be used.

BASIC VAGINAL INSTRUMENTS (FIG. 4)

- Scalpel handle, solid, straight no. 3—1, no. 4L—1; surgical blades as per choice
- Sponge holding/Dressing forceps, standard 14.5 cm—1, standard 20 cm—1
- Tissue forceps, 1 × 2 teeth 14.5 cm and 18 cm—1 each, 25 cm—6 nos
- *Kelly hemostatic forceps/artery forceps:* 14 cm, straight 4 and curved 4 each
- *Vulsellum:* Single or multiple jaw
- *Retractors:* Deaver, Jayle's self-retaining, Heaney's, Soonawalla's, Sims anterior vaginal wall, etc.
- *Speculums:* Sims, Cusco, Auvard, etc.
- Uterine sound and set of dilators, curettes
- Myoma Screw
- *Needle holder:* Small and standard
- Sponges, suction cannula
- Suture materials as per requirements
- Mesh if required

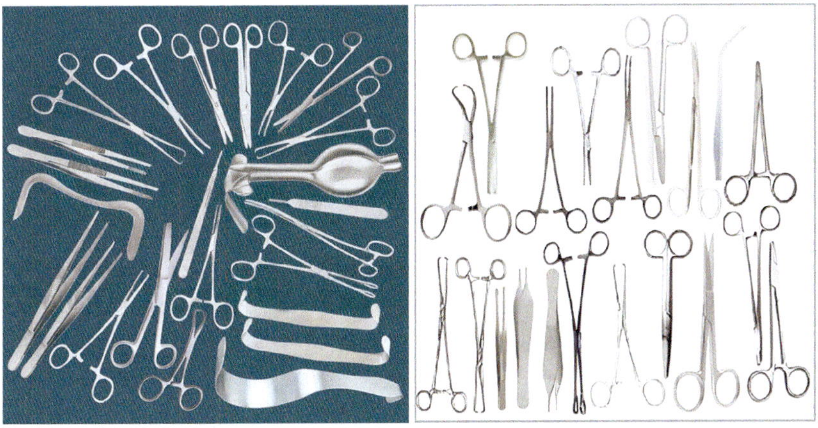

Fig. 4: Basic vaginal instruments.

- Urinary bladder catheter, Foley's no. 14 FG
- Sterile drapings and sheets
- *Diathermy:* Monopolar, Bipolar
- *Different sealing devices:* LigaSure provides a combination of pressure and energy to create vessel fusion.
    i. Permanently fuses vessels up to and including 7 mm in diameter and tissue bundles without dissection or isolation
    ii. Average seal cycle is 2–4 seconds, when used with the Force Triad™ energy platform
    iii. Seals withstand three times normal systolic blood pressure
    iv. Feedback-controlled response system automatically discontinues energy delivery when the seal cycle is complete, eliminating the guesswork

Biclamp with local vessel sealers, principle is approximately same as LigaSure, locally made, reusable unlimited times and very cheap.

Benefits of Biclamp and Vessel Sealer

- The length and shape of biclamp jaws is adapted to the body; target tissue can be reached even with reduced surgical access.
- Steel coating of jaws prevents tissues from sticking to forceps and carbonization.
- Effective sealing of 2–7 mm vessels in seconds (usually 2–4 sec) by coagulating tissue structures over larger areas by melting collagen and elastin in vessel wall to form a seal zone, without producing any charred foreign material due to autostop function of machine. Surgery is virtually bloodless and ultrafast recovery follows.
- Ceramic insulated jaws reduce the risk of lateral thermal damage to adjacent tissues and structures.
- Reusable biclamps save disposables and suture materials' cost, less operating room time and less medication.
- Individual dissection of vessels is not necessary, and patient does not get any current. Absence of tissue necrosis and foreign bodies (including sutures) results in reduction of resorption process and phagocytosis thereby reducing postoperative pain. Thermal burns of skin, mucosa and ureter are to be avoided.

Harmonic: The harmonic scalpel is a surgical instrument that (unlike electrosurgery) uses ultrasonic vibrations (55,000 Hz) to cut and cauterize tissue. The harmonic scalpel may be superior to electrosurgery in that it can cut through thicker tissue, creates less toxic surgical smoke, and poses somewhat less of a risk for electrocution or other potentially fatal complications.

Lasers: Needed for different cutting, coagulation, rejuvenation as per choice and need of surgeon.

CONCLUSION

ACOG strongly favors vaginal hysterectomy wherever feasible compared to trans-abdominal or laparoscopic or robotic approach. Vaginal natural orifice transluminal endoscopic surgery (vNOTES) is gradually becoming popular. A faulty surgeon quarrels with instruments. Requirements of instruments and facilities take a back seat with increasing experience and confidence. There is no end to advancement, but reasonable facilities should facilitate reasonable completion of procedures in a satisfactory manner. Thus, we serve our patients with the utmost care in a nice way.

To complete non-descent vaginal hysterectomy (NDVH): Under regional anesthesia, Only 2 artery forceps, one Jayle's self-retaining retractor, one ampoule of V-Press, one 50 mL injection syringe with needle, 200 mL of sterile normal saline, one kidney dish, one bladder retractor, one Soonawalla"s speculum, 2 hysterectomy clamps, one needle holder, suction cannula, one mop, vessel sealer and one 70 cm no 0-vicryl should suffice. With experience and positivity, contraindications become indications for surgery.

6 CHAPTER

Sutures, Needles and Suturing Techniques

Suman Sinha, Niharika Allu

INTRODUCTION

The primary objective of suturing is to obtain adequate closure of the wound (skin, subcutaneous tissue, fascia, visceral organs) to enhance healing. It can only be achieved by having a good knowledge of the various suture materials and needles available in the market and knowing where to use what and applying the apt suturing technique for that wound. This chapter endeavors to give you a brief outline of the various sutures, types of needles and common suturing techniques which are used in daily practice.

SUTURES

Sutures which are easy to use by the surgeon, have good tensile strength, are inexpensive, cause minimal tissue reaction and easily visible are the ideal sutures. But most of the sutures have one or two of these characteristics missing. Sutures can be classified based on three different characteristics:[1]

1. Absorbable vs. non-absorbable **(Table 1)**
2. Natural vs. synthetic **(Table 2)**
3. Monofilament vs. multifilament **(Table 3)**

TABLE 1: Absorbable vs. non-absorbable.

Absorbable Sutures	*Non-absorbable sutures*
Lose their tensile strength over a period of time from few weeks to months	Do not lose their tensile strength with time
Used for deeper tissues, e.g., uterine closure, etc.	Used for permanent ligation or long-term closures, e.g., vessel ligation, hernia, fascial closure
For superficial tissues, use rapid absorbable sutures to avoid scarring, e.g., polyglactin 910 (Vicryl), polydioxanone (PDS), poliglecaprone (Monocryl)	Need to be removed if used for superficial tissues like skin, e.g., Nylon, polypropylene (Prolene)

TABLE 2: Natural vs. synthetic.

Natural sutures	*Synthetic sutures*
• Obtained from purified animal tissues • External serosa of bovine intestines e.g., catgut, chromic catgut, silk	Manmade, e.g., polypropylene, nylon, PDS, poliglecaprone (monocryl), polyglactin 910 (Vicryl)
Degrades by proteolysis (absorbable)—causes more inflammation	Degrades by hydrolysis—causes less inflammation

TABLE 3: Monofilament vs. multifilament.

Monofilament sutures	*Multifilament sutures*
Single filament, less surface area	Braided or twisted
Higher memory, difficult to handle, need more knots	Less memory, more pliable
Pass easily through tissues	More friction through tissues
Less inflammation	More inflammation, more chances of infection
Less expensive	More expensive – impregnated with antibiotics, coated for easy gliding
e.g., nylon, polypropylene (prolene), polydioxanone (PDS)	e.g., polyglactin 910 (Vicryl), silk

Sutures are numbered by their thickness. Sutures numbered 0-10 are thick, with increasing thickness with each number. Sutures numbered 1-0 to 12-0 are thinner sutures with higher numbers preceding the zero denoting the thinnest suture.

Barbed sutures are also available which can be used for knotless suturing even in subcuticular tissues as they distribute the tension across the wound and cause bidirectional fixation of the wound and give better cosmesis.[2]

NEEDLES

There are three parts of a needle—eye, body, and point. Suture can be swagged onto the needle as is the case with most modern sutures or threaded through the eye. The shape of the needle can be straight or curved. Curved needles can be 1/4, 1/2, 3/8 or 1/3 of a circle **(Fig. 1)**.[3]

- *Cutting—conventional* (cutting edge on the inner side of the needle—used for tough tissues)/*reverse cutting* (cutting edge on the outer side of needle—to reduce risk of tissue cutout).
- *Tapered* (rounded)—*sharp* (punctures and then dilates the tissues)/ *blunt* (spreads rather than cuts the tissue-softer tissues).

There is no set rule for which suture and needle should be used where but clinical scenario should be taken into view to enhance faster healing and

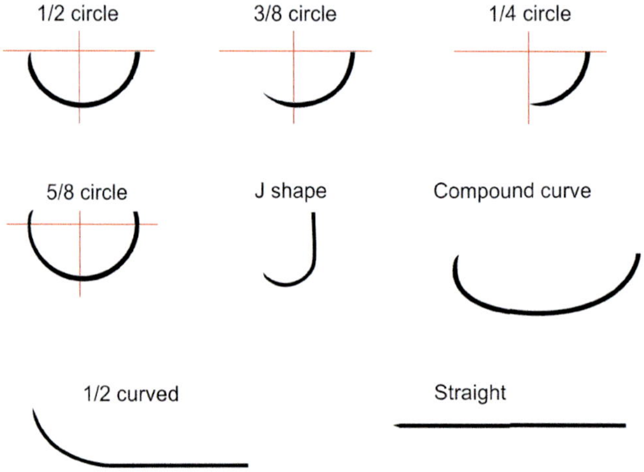

Fig. 1: Needle tip.

to cause less morbidity to the patients. For example, avoid multifilament sutures when risk of infection is high, use non-absorbable sutures for closure of hernia, absorbable sutures for faster healing tissues like viscera, cosmesis for skin wound can be achieved by using smaller poliglecaprone (Monocryl) if subcuticular suturing technique is employed.[1]

Meticulous handling of the sutures during knotting and avoiding holding with instruments and avoiding undue pressure on the suture is essential for preventing damage and premature breakdown of the sutures.[4]

SUTURING TECHNIQUES

The surgical technique used to close a given wound depends on the force and direction of tensions on the wound. Wound closure techniques now range from simple sutures to adhesive compounds and techniques have also improved. Perfect suture approximation and wound care are extremely important in regenerative methods.[5,7]

Objective

- Closing dead space
- Provide adequate tension
- Provide support to tissues
- Approximate skin edges
- Promote healing
- Maintain hemostasis
- Reduce pain
- Prevent infection

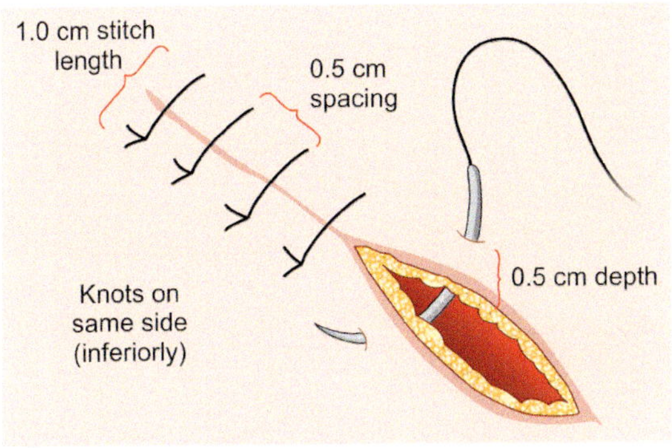

Fig. 2: Simple interrupted suture.

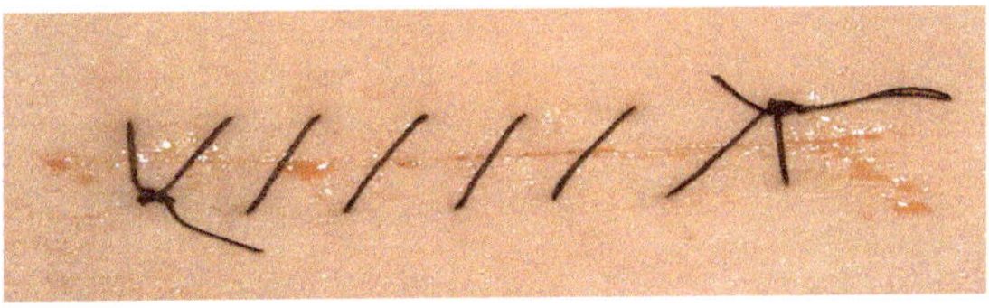

Fig. 3: Simple running suture.

Types of Suturing Techniques

Simple Interrupted Suture

This technique is usually applied to simple wounds both traumatic and surgical. The suture is placed by inserting the needle perpendicular to the tissue 3–5 mm away from the edge, traversing the full thickness of the tissue and exiting perpendicular to the tissue on the opposite side, the stitch should be wider at the base **(Fig. 2)**. It needs to be repeated depending on the wound length and the sutures should be placed 0.5 cm apart.[6]

Advantages: Easy to place, has greater tensile strength, less potential for causing wound edema and impaired cutaneous circulation.

Disadvantages: Increased length of time required for placement, greater risk of crosshatched suture lines.

Simple Running Suture

A simple running suture is essentially an uninterrupted series of simple interrupted sutures **(Fig. 3)**. A series of simple interrupted stitches are placed in succession without the suture material being tied or cut after each pass. The suture should be evenly placed, and tension should be evenly distributed along the suture line. The line of stitches is completed by tying a knot after the last pass.

Advantages: Quicker placement, rapid approximation of wounds.

Disadvantages: Risk of dehiscence, puckering of stitches if placed in thin skin.

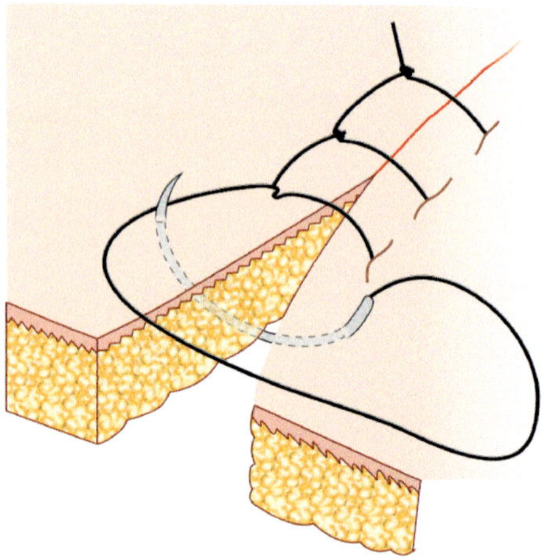

Fig. 4: Running locked suture.

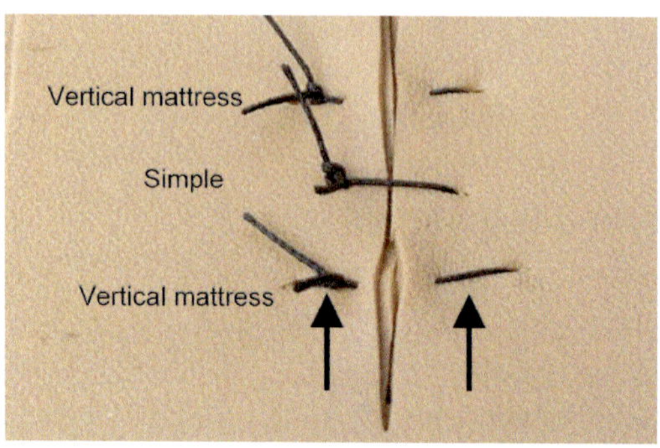

Fig. 5: Vertical mattress suture.

Running Locked Suture

The traditional running suture is locked by passing the needle through the loop preceding it as each stitch is placed **(Fig. 4)**.

Advantages: Increased tensile strength, useful in wounds requiring additional hemostasis.

Disadvantages: Increased risk of impairing microcirculation surrounding the wound, can cause tissue strangulation if placed too tightly.

Vertical Mattress Suture

It consists of simple interrupted stitch placed wide and deep into the wound edge and a second interrupted stitch is placed close to the wound edge and in the opposite direction. The width of the stitch is increased in proportion to the amount of tension on the wound **(Fig. 5)**.

Advantages: Maximum wound eversion, reduces dead space, minimizes wound tension.

Disadvantage: Cross-hatching is greater because of 4 entry points of the stitch.

Horizontal Mattress Suture

The horizontal mattress suture is placed by entering the skin 5 mm to 1 cm from the wound edge, the suture is then passed deep into the dermis to the opposite side of the suture line and exits the skin equidistant from the wound edge, the needle re-enters the skin on the same side 5 mm to 1 cm lateral to the exit point, the stitch is passed deep to the opposite side of the wound, where it exits the skin and the knot is tied **(Fig. 6)**.

Advantages: Useful for wounds under high tension may be used as a stay stitch to temporarily approximate wound.

Disadvantages: Risk of producing scar marks if left for longer than 7 days, risk of tissue strangulation if tied too tightly.

Running Subcuticular Stitches

The running subcuticular sutures is placed by taking horizontal bites through the papillary dermis on alternating side of the wound. No suture is visible, and suture may be left in place for several weeks **(Fig. 7)**.

Advantages: Good cosmetic result, eliminate cross-hatching.

Disadvantages: Does not provide wound strength, require precise approximation of wound edges.

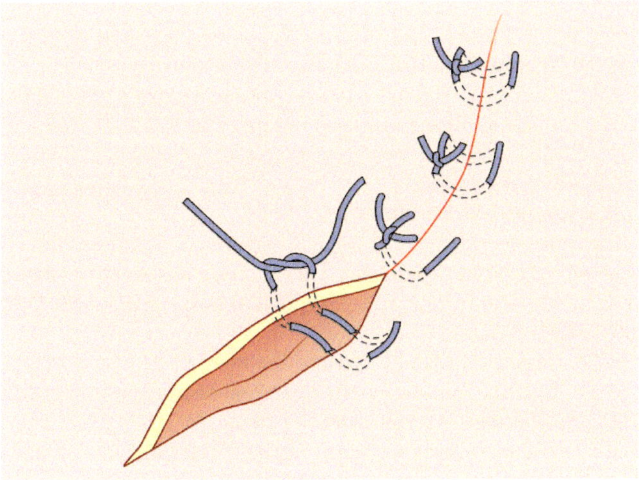

Fig. 6: Horizontal mattress suture.

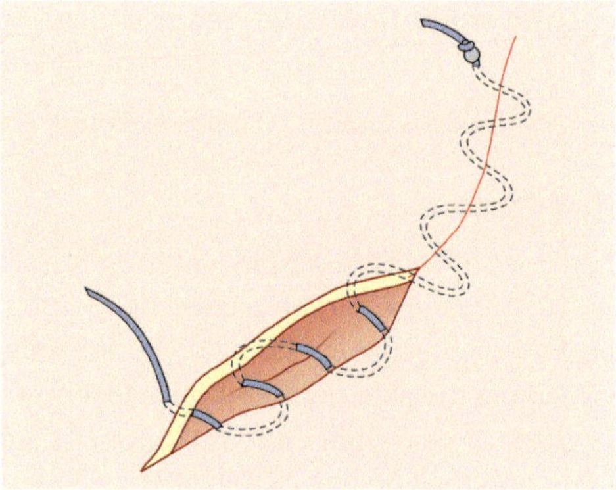

Fig. 7: Running subcuticular stitches.

Knot Tying Technique

Once the suture is properly placed, it should be secured with a knot. The square knot is traditionally used. The tip of the needle holder is rotated clockwise around the long end of the suture for two complete turns then with the tip of the needle holder catch holds the tail end of the suture and pulls through the loops of the long end and tied to approximate the wound edges without constricting the tissue.

CONCLUSION

In-depth knowledge of various characteristics of sutures and needles and knowing the different suturing techniques of wound closure by the surgeons and the nursing staff helps in giving quality care to the patients in each clinical scenarios.

REFERENCES

1. Rose J, Tuma F. Sutures and needles. [Updated 2023 Aug 28]. In: Stat Pearls [Internet]. Treasure Island (FL): Stat Pearls Publishing; 2024 Jan.
2. Tripathi K, Tiwari VK, Sinha A, Sharma MK. Skin closure with barbed sutures: an early evaluation of cosmesis and complications. J Head Neck Spine Surg. 2021;4(4):555643. doi: 10.19080/JHNSS.2021.04.555643.
3. Byrne M, Aly A. The surgical needle. Aesthet Surg J. 2019;39(Suppl_2):S73-7. doi: 10.1093/asj/sjz035. PMID: 30869752.
4. Polykandriotis E, Daenicke J, Bolat A, Grüner J, Schubert DW, Horch RE. Individualized wound closure-mechanical properties of suture materials. J Pers Med. 2022;12(7):1041. doi: 10.3390/jpm12071041. PMID: 35887538; PMCID: PMC9316899.
5. Azmat CE, Council M. Wound Closure Techniques. [Updated 2023 Jun 26]. In: Stat Pearls [Internet]. Treasure Island (FL): Stat Pearls Publishing; 2024 Jan.
6. Stoecker A, Blattner CM, Howerter S, Fancher W, Young J, Lear W. Effect of simple interrupted suture spacing on aesthetic and functional outcomes of skin closure. J Cutan Med Surgery. 2019;23(6):580-5.
7. Suturing skills e-Book—Dr Marshall Murdoch, Jan 2015.

CHAPTER 7

Use of Single Bladed Vaginal Speculum with Light Source for Non-descent Vaginal Hysterectomy and Posterior Perineorrhaphy

Sucheta Hiray-Bachhav, Asavari Karani

Vaginal surgery would be impossible without the use of the speculum. The most common one used in practice is the Sims speculum invented by the Father of Gynecology, American gynecologist J Marion Sims (1813–1883).

It is omnipresent in vaginal surgeries from episiotomy repair, anterior and posterior perineorrhaphy, vaginal hysterectomy to aesthetic procedures like Vaginal reconstruction, Vaginoplasty, Labiaplasty, Valvopathy, Vaginal rejuvenation, Clitoral hood reduction and a Perineoplasty **(Fig. 1)**.

The vagina is an elastic muscular tube of 7–10 cm in length that extends from the vulva (female external genitalia) to the cervix of the uterus where it ends in an anterior and posterior fornix. The vaginal canal is positioned between the urethra and bladder anteriorly, and the rectum posteriorly. The vaginal opening is in the posterior portion of the vulvar vestibule, behind the urethral opening. It is surrounded on either side by the labia minora medially and labia majora laterally.[1]

Proper exposure and retraction of this muscular organ during vaginal surgery can be quite challenging especially in younger non-parous women who have not yet undergone pregnancy and childbirth. Often, multiple

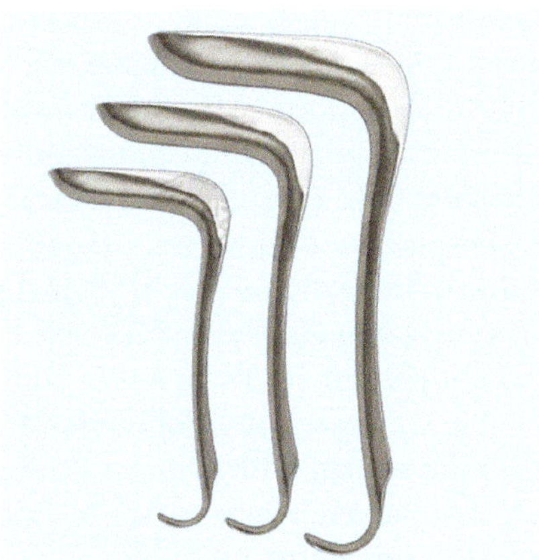

Fig. 1: Sims speculum.

assistants are required on either side of surgeons restricting the maneuvering surgically as well as obstruction of illumination of vagina via external light source.

The external force applied for retraction for adequate visualization for surgical accuracy can often cause vaginal and labial tears and injuries, which can be deleterious in patients, especially one who is undergoing aesthetic surgery.

Obstetric vaginal lacerations and cervical tears can also be extremely challenging in cases of difficult or instrumental deliveries where proper exposure and visualization of apex of laceration can be challenging in a patient who is actively bleeding from the wound and time is of essence to repair the injury and secure hemostasis.[2]

In this backdrop, Quinn et al., introduced a single-bladed speculum with a light source similar to a laryngoscope for vaginal examination. It helped greatly in ease of vaginal surgery especially with patients with a narrow vagina.[3]

Non-descent vaginal hysterectomy (NDVH) although recommended by ACOG,[4] for non-prolapsed uteri 12 weeks or lesser in size as the preferred method of hysterectomy, has very less takers as newly passed out gynecologists believe that it takes more effort, time and surgical expertise as compared to the abdominal or laparoscopic route. The laparoscopic route has a steep-learning curve, increased operative time and is associated with increased rate of injuries to bowel, bladder and ureters in previously operated case or those with dense adhesions due to endometriosis or pelvic inflammatory disease.[5]

Patients undergoing abdominal hysterectomy in hospitals with a lack of access to the instruments and expertise required for laparoscopic surgery have an increased postoperative recovery time and a greater incidence of postoperative morbidity due to longer hospitalization.[5]

The common belief that bigger, bulky uteri, endometriosis, pelvic inflammatory disease, previous surgeries,[6] and narrow vagina make vaginal hysterectomy difficult to be performed are not considered to be contraindications for non-descent vaginal hysterectomy and can be successfully attempted in all these conditions **(Fig. 2)**. It has a clear advantage over the abdominal route in obese women.[7] However, proper selection of patients is a critical factor in determining the success of vaginal procedures. Lack of expertise and the curve in learning the technique also has major impact on the number of procedures performed. The possible complications of NDVH include bleeding of cut and ligated stumps of uterine artery, bladder injury while dissection of anterior pouch, vault hematoma, urinary tract infection, fever, sepsis due to pelvic hematoma.[8] In such a situation, using single-bladed light source speculum which takes up less space than a double-bladed speculum, requires less traction and is easy to maneuver in a narrow

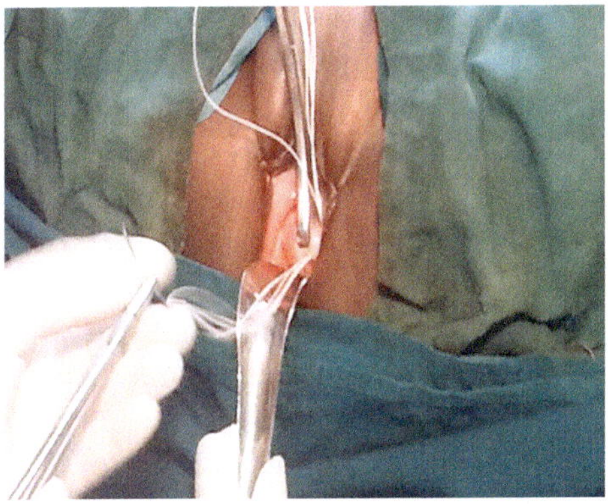

Fig. 2: Surgery photograph.

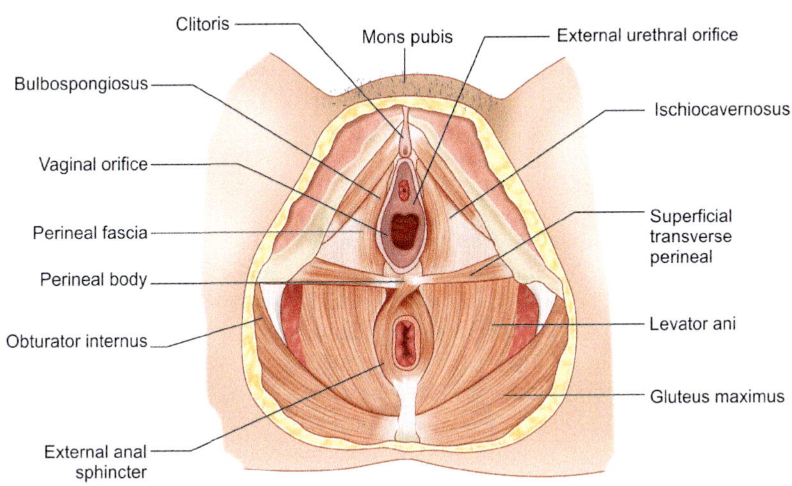

Fig. 3: Perineal body anatomy.

vagina in a patient undergoing NDVH has massive benefits in vision and ease of surgery. It will take away the apprehension of vaginal surgeries in non-prolapsed uteri and re-introduce vaginal hysterectomy as the first surgical option in those posted for hysterectomy.

Perineorrhaphy and perineoplasty is performed for prevention of recurrent prolapse, improved sexual function, treatment of pain and cosmesis.

Female genital cosmetic surgery (FGCS) is one of the fastest growing areas in aesthetic plastic surgery **(Fig. 3)**.[9] When performed in the appropriate patients, FGCS procedures have high satisfaction and low complication rates.[10]

Many women after a single or multiple vaginal delivery may experience vaginal laxity due to local tissue stretching and separation of the pelvic floor musculature. Women may complain of altered sexual satisfaction and a generalized feeling of laxity.[11] Women also commonly complain of gaping of the vaginal vestibule, which creates an aesthetic deformity allowing visibility of the vaginal mucosa. This gaping also creates several functional concerns including altered ability to achieve orgasm, and vaginal air entrapment resulting in embarrassing sounds during sexual intercourse.[12]

Since cosmetic perineoplasty is offered in many clinics all over the country, it is highly desirable to introduce an instrument which can make this now ubiquitous procedure easier on the clinician and make the surgery more efficient.

The potential complications of perineoplasty are bleeding, hematoma, infection, wound dehiscence, urinary retention, injury to bowel/bladder, development of a rectovaginal fistula, scarring, vaginal stenosis, dyspareunia, altered sensation, and an inadequate surgical outcome in terms of patient satisfaction.[13]

Usage of the correct instruments during the surgery will go a long way in preventing and reducing the rate of complications during surgery and improve postoperative patient satisfaction.

REFERENCES

1. Gold JM, Shrimanker I. Physiology, Vaginal. 2023 Jul 24. In: StatPearls [Internet]. Treasure Island (FL): StatPearls Publishing; 2024 Jan–. PMID: 31424731.
2. Ramar CN, Vadakekut ES, Grimes WR. Perineal Lacerations. [Updated 2024 Aug 11]. In: StatPearls [Internet]. Treasure Island (FL): StatPearls Publishing; 2024 Jan-. Available from: https://www.ncbi.nlm.nih.gov/books/NBK559068/
3. Quinn MJ. An illuminated vaginal speculum. Am J Obstet Gynecol. 1999;180(1 Pt 1): 33-4. doi: 10.1016/s0002-9378(99)70145-6. PMID: 9914574.
4. American College of Obstetricians and Gynecologists. ACOG Committee Opinion. Number 311, April 2005. Appropriate use of laparoscopically assisted vaginal hysterectomy. Obstet Gynecol. 2005;105(4):929-30. doi: 10.1097/00006250-200504000-00059. PMID: 15802439.
5. Umeora OUJ, Onoh RC, Eze JN, Igberase GO. Abdominal versus vaginal hysterectomy: appraisal of indications and complications in a Nigerian Federal Medical Centre. Nep Journ OG. 2009;4(1):25-9.
6. Coulam CB, Pratt JH. Vaginal hysterectomy: is previous pelvic operation a contraindication? Am J Obstet Gynecol. 1973;116(2):252-60. doi: 10.1016/0002-9378(73)91060-0. PMID: 4712423.
7. Pitkin RM. Vaginal hysterectomy in obese women. Obstet Gynecol. 1977;49(5):567-9. PMID: 850571.
8. Sarada Murali M, Khan A. A comparative study of non-descent vaginal hysterectomy and laparoscopic hysterectomy. J Obstet Gynaecol India. 2019;69(4):369-73. doi: 10.1007/s13224-019-01227-1. Epub 2019 Apr 27. PMID: 31391746; PMCID: PMC6661041.
9. Cosmetic Surgery National Data Bank Statistics. Aesthet Surg J. 2018;38(suppl 3): 1-24. doi: 10.1093/asj/sjy132. PMID: 29846503.

10. Barbara G, Facchin F, Buggio L, Alberico D, Frattaruolo MP, Kustermann A. Vaginal rejuvenation: current perspectives. Int J Womens Health. 2017;9:513-9. doi: 10.2147/IJWH.S99700. PMID: 28860864; PMCID: PMC5560421.
11. Ulubay M, Keskin U, Fidan U, Ozturk M, Bodur S, Yılmaz A, Kinci MF, Yenen MC. Safety, efficiency, and outcomes of perineoplasty: treatment of the sensation of a wide vagina. Biomed Res Int. 2016;2016:2495105. doi: 10.1155/2016/2495105. Epub 2016 Aug 17. PMID: 27610368; PMCID: PMC5005521.
12. Ostrzenski A. Modified posterior perineoplasty in women. J Reprod Med. 2015;60(3-4):109-16. PMID: 25898473.
13. Goodman MP, Placik OJ, Benson RH 3rd, Miklos JR, Moore RD, Jason RA, Matlock DL, Simopoulos AF, Stern BH, Stanton RA, Kolb SE, Gonzalez F. A large multicenter outcome study of female genital plastic surgery. J Sex Med. 2010;7(4 Pt 1):1565-77. doi: 10.1111/j.1743-6109.2009.01573.x. Epub 2009 Nov 12. PMID: 19912495.

8

CHAPTER

Surgical Anatomy of the Pelvis: As Applicable for Vaginal Hysterectomy

Rajkumar H Shah

The uterus is a unique organ as it lies suspended in the pelvic cavity, by its elastic supports. These supports allow the uterus to get distended during pregnancy and involute back to its original location. These supports require to be cut, and transfixed whenever surgery for its removal is done. These supports are enumerated here:

- *Upper tier supports:*
  1. The round ligaments
  2. Broad ligament with intervening pelvic cellular tissues
  3. Endopelvic fascia covering the uterus
- *Middle tier supports:*
  1. Cervicovaginal junction—important direct support (fibromuscular tissue surrounding the vessels and nerves)
  2. Pelvic cellular tissues (connective tissue and smooth muscles) through which blood vessels and nerve supply pass through from lateral pelvic wall, condense surrounding them and give direct support.
  3. The condensation of the tissues surrounding the supravaginal cervix and vagina down to the superior layer of the fascia covering the cervicovaginal junction.
  4. The condensation and reinforcement by plain muscles to form ligaments—Mackenrodt's, uterosacral and pubocervical.
- Inferior tier

Musculofascial tone of the hollow vagina by the fascial condensation at the vault and by the pelvic floor.

The uterus and its supports are covered by the visceral peritoneum which gets reflected anteriorly from the roof of the bladder on to the anterior abdominal wall forming the parietal peritoneum and posteriorly on to the rectum reaching lower into the pelvis forming the cul-de-sac (pouch of Douglas). At hysterectomy, once these pouches are rendered open, the blood supply to the uterus can be approached, on the lateral aspects **(Fig. 1)**.

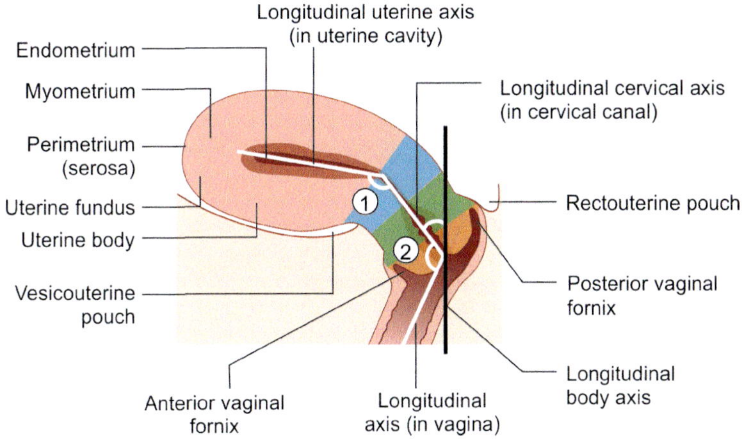

Fig. 1: Surgical anatomy of the pelvis.

BLOOD SUPPLY OF THE UTERUS

Whenever, a surgical extirpation of an organ is planned, it is imperative to know the intricacies of its blood supply. The uterus is no exception. In fact, when a vaginal hysterectomy is done for a bulky uterus, there are ways and means of morcellation of the uterus and at this point in time, knowing the blood supply of the uterus is very important **(Fig. 2)**.

The blood supply is mainly from:

- The uterine artery, arising as a branch of the internal iliac artery and then dividing into the ascending and descending branch.
- The ovarian artery arising from the aorta, and anastomosing with the ascending uterine, within the broad ligament.

The ascending uterine artery gives off arcuate vessels at regular intervals from the lateral walls to the midline and joins up with other vessels from the opposite side. This makes the midline least vascular **(Fig. 3)**.

In view of the blood supply arising from both sides, it is essential to go symmetrically to impede the blood vessels by use of clamps or sutures and prevent blood loss.

It is essential to deliver the fundus of the uterus from the anterior pouch, to maintain the anatomical relations. If delivered from the posterior pouch, the normal anatomy could get distorted, but can still be done at times, if deemed necessary.

APPLIED SURGICAL ANATOMY

The incision on the cervix anteriorly has to be planned to avoid injury to the urinary bladder. Especially, in prolapse uterus, too low an incision would result in unnecessary extensive dissection before reaching the anterior

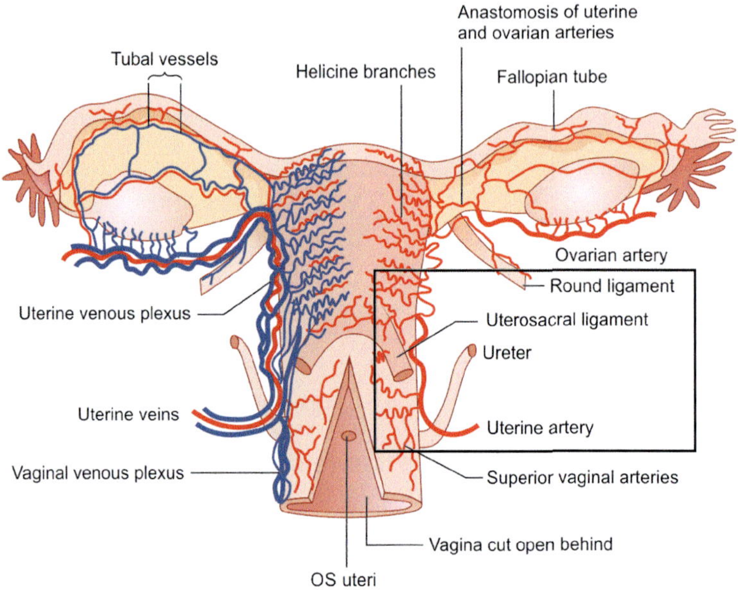

Fig. 2: Blood supply of the uterus.

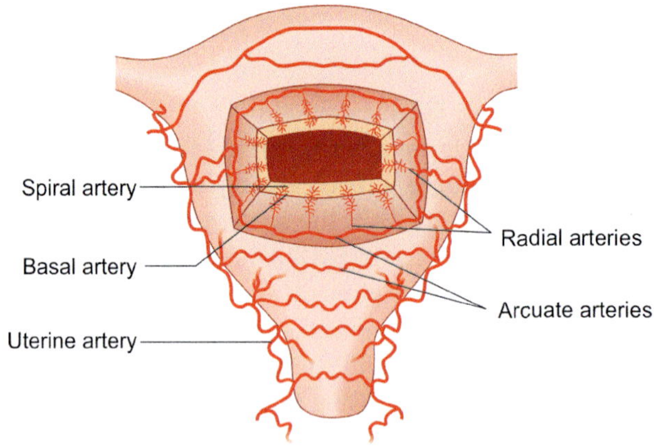

Fig. 3: Ascending uterine artery.

pouch. A very high incision may be easier to approach the anterior pouch but may lead to sacrificing a large portion of the vagina, compromising the effective length of the vagina leading to sexual problems postsurgery.

The anterior pouch can be rendered open in three simple steps. First, placing the anterior incision on the cervix. Second, sharp dissection and picking up the vesicouterine ligament. This can be incised, exposing the anterior pouch. Third, picking up the peritoneum between two hemostats and incising the peritoneum to render the anterior pouch open.

The posterior incision is taken in different ways. An Ellis forceps could be placed on the posterior vaginal wall, grasping the underlying peritoneum of the pouch and opening it in one swift incision with a scissors. The only disadvantage of this method is that it compromises a large portion of the vagina, reducing its effective length. A second method would be to do it identical to the anterior pouch, by incising the vagina and dissecting till the posterior peritoneum is reached and then incising it between two Ellis forceps. This maintains a decent length of the vagina, but could cause bleeding due to excessive dissection, once the effect of injected adrenaline solution wears off.

Once, both the pouches are opened, it is essential to apply clamps or place sutures in such a manner that both the leaves of the broad ligament are included, so as to take care of all the branches of the uterine artery.

When a bulky uterus is being delivered vaginally, there are various ways the uterus is morcellated—bisection or decompressing by Lash's technique. These involve clamping and ligating the uterine arteries and then proceeding with the morcellation procedure. Once the uterine arteries are obliterated, the morcellation procedure becomes almost bloodless.

Lastly, if the adnexa is to be excised, the proximal part of the infundibulopelvic ligament is identified and special clamps applied before excision.

It is essential to maintain a good length of the vagina at surgery, for allowing satisfactory coital function, postsurgery. This can be done by adhering to the suggestions made above as also, suspending the vault of the vagina to the adnexal stumps.

SUGGESTED READING

1. Chung KW. Gross Anatomy, 4th edition. Philadelphia Lippincott Williams & Wilkins; 2000.
2. De Lancy JOL. The Anatomy of the pelvic floor. Curr Opin Obstet Gynecol1994.
3. De Lancy JOL. What's new in the functional anatomy of pelvic organ prolapse? Curr Opin Obstet Gynecol. 2016;28(5):420-9.
4. Gray H. Anatomy, Descriptive and Surgical, The Unabridged Gray's Anatomy. Philadelphia: Running Press, 1999.
5. Handa VL, Van Le L. Te Linde's Operative Gynecology. 12th edition; 2019.
6. Katz VL, Lentz GM, Lobo RA, Gershenson DM. Comprehensive Gynecology 5th edition. Philadelphia: Mosby Elsevier, 2007.
7. Miller Ashton JA, De Lancey JOL. Functional anatomy of the pelvic floor. Ann N Y Acad Sci. 2007;1101;266-96.
8. Standring S. Gray's Anatomy: The Anatomical Basis of Clinical Practice, 42nd edition; 2021, Chapter 22-23.

9 CHAPTER

Prevention of Bladder and Ureteric Injuries in Obs-Gyn Practice

T Srikala Prasad

INTRODUCTION

The female reproductive tract and urinary tract are intimately related anatomically. Common clinical conditions like previous lower segment cesarean section (LSCS), previous pelvic surgeries, endometriosis, adhesions, cervical fibroid, broad ligament fibroid, procidentia, malignancy, excessive intraoperative bleeding and placenta accreta spectrum disorder, lead to altered anatomy which makes the patient at increased risk of urological surgeries during OB-GYN interventions.[1,2] The majority of such injuries occur during cesarean section and hysterectomy.[2]

A good history taking, dedicated clinical examination, and appropriate investigations will help us identify women at risk for urological injuries.

The first step in the prevention of bladder injury is to catheterize the bladder. A distended bladder is more prone to inadvertent injury. Good anatomical knowledge, surgical expertise, good exposure, adequate lighting, effective help from assistants, and necessary equipment is essential for a good surgery.

SPECIFIC PREVENTIVE MEASURES DURING LSCS AND ABDOMINAL SURGERIES

We need to exert care while we operate on a patient who has undergone prior surgeries as the bladder may be drawn up and present at the site of the incision itself. While opening the peritoneum, we need to ensure that we are opening only the leaves of the peritoneum and there is nothing beneath it. It may be even better to open more cranially **(Fig. 1)**.

Opening the UV fold of peritoneum is normally a simple procedure. In case of patients who have had previous LSCS, there can be morbid adhesion of the bladder to the lower uterine segment. Careful sharp dissection will help us to safely mobilize the bladder. In repeat LSCS patients, bladder injuries most commonly occur during three specific steps. First, when creating the bladder flap, injuries happen in 43–60% of cases. Next, injuries can occur while entering the peritoneal cavity, which happens in 30–33% of cases. Finally, during the incision or delivery, injuries occur in 10–24% of cases **(Fig. 2)**.[3]

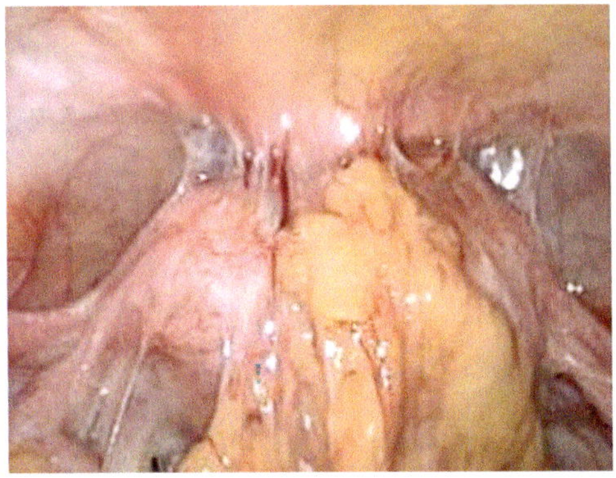

Fig. 1: Dense bladder adhesions in the case of previous LSCS.

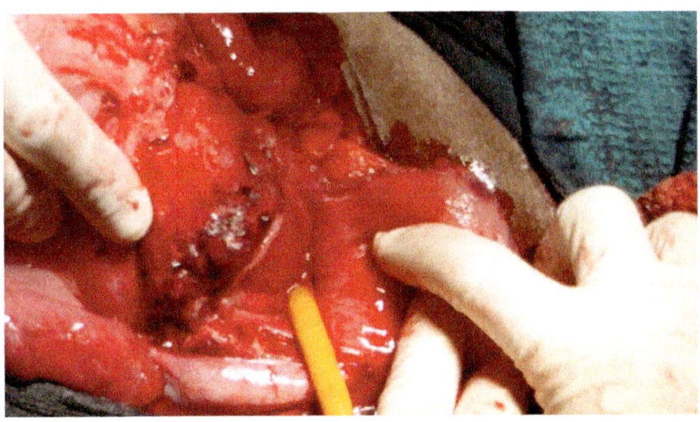

Fig. 2: Anterior wall of the bladder is mobilized. The posterior wall is morbidly adherent to the lower uterine segment and bladder found opened.

For a patient with a deeply engaged head during LSCS, it is preferable to deliver as breech, use Patwardhan's maneuver, or put an inverted T-shaped incision. This will avoid inadvertent extension of the uterine incision leading to retroperitoneal hematoma. In such a situation, we need to open the broad ligament carefully (beware of the ureter which may cling on to the medial leaf of the peritoneum), remove any clots present and safely achieve hemostasis. It is imperative that blind clamping must not be done to secure hemostasis. If done, it may lead to ureteric injuries which are otherwise rare in obstetric practice.

SPECIAL CARE IN PLACENTA ACCRETA SPECTRUM DISORDER (FIG. 3)

Emergency surgery can be demanding, especially doing LSCS in placenta accreta spectrum (PAS) where the lower uterine segment is enlarged and vascular.[3] There is distortion of normal anatomy, possible placental invasion

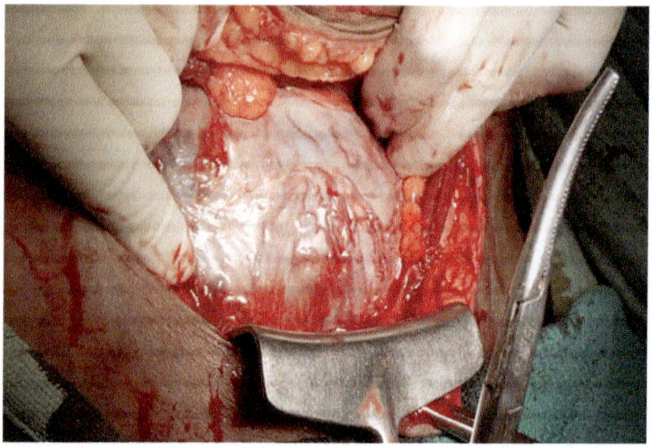

Fig. 3: Placenta percreta with threatened rupture.

and there is profuse bleeding. It is better to operate on these patients in a well-equipped facility with adequate blood, skilled assistants and alerts given to urologists. The family needs to be extensively counseled regarding the possible complications including the need for an obstetric hysterectomy.

Performing subtotal hysterectomy is not a risk factor for developing ureteric injury. If the need arises for doing a hysterectomy as in the case of PAS, we need to do a total hysterectomy with the possibility of inadvertent bladder and ureteric injuries (overall injuries were 21.7%, with bladder injuries at 11.7%, ureter at 4.7%, and bladder with ureter at 5.3%).[4] Dallas et al. found a four times higher rate of genitourinary injury in the women who needed obstetric hysterectomy.[5]

Prevention of Bladder Injuries in Incontinence Surgeries

- Follow the guidelines
- Empty bladder is protective
- Transobturator taping has less chance of bladder injury compared to retropubic.
- *Intraoperative check cystoscopy* can diagnose inadvertent bladder injury. The needle can be retrieved, and carefully reinserted and check cystoscopy is done.
- No need for any formal repair.
- Bladder to be decompressed with a continuous Foley's catheter for 10 days.

Specific Preventive Measures during Vaginal Surgeries

In cases of long-standing, irreducible procidentia with bilateral gross hydroureteronephrosis may be seen in up to 40%, the ureters are often grossly dilated and tortuous and are dragged down looking like the knee of the ureter.[6] *Pessary placement* for a few weeks will make the POP surgery simpler and reduce the chances of inadvertent ureteric injury.

Emptying the bladder prior to any vaginal procedure is an important step in preventing bladder injury. The next step is to correctly open the anterior pouch. Hydrodissection will facilitate the dissection. The circular incision on the vaginal wall is placed at the bladder sulcus which marks the junction of the bladder to the anterior vaginal wall. We can also see the sulcus when we lift the anterior vaginal wall with our non-dominant hand or lift by applying Allis forceps and give traction with Vulsellum applied to the anterior lip of the cervix. The bladder sulcus can be seen as a crease in the anterior vaginal wall when we give a slight inward push to the cervix.

Traction applied to the anterior lip of the cervix and counter traction by the allis forceps on the anterior vaginal overlying the bladder will guide us in determining the appropriate depth of the circular incision till it reaches the cervical stroma. The bladder can be safely mobilized by cutting the bladder pillars, eventually reaching and opening the anterior peritoneal reflection. A retractor placed here will safely push the bladder and ureters away. The principle of using sharp dissection and following Sheth's lateral window can be used in cases where there is morbid adhesion following previous LSCS.[4] A clear urine drained now not only empties the bladder but also is reassuring that there has been no bladder injury.

URETERIC INJURY

Dallas et al. in their study done in California have noticed an interesting observation that Asian women had the highest rate of genitourinary injury during hysterectomy, possibly because they also had the highest rates of endometriosis.[5]

Causes of Ureteric Injury

Intraoperative ureteric injury can be caused by crushing or clamping inadvertently, suture ligation, avulsion, complete or partial transection, or injury due to devascularization (which can happen during Wertheim's hysterectomy).

The ureter can be damaged by the lateral spread of heat from the energy sources used during laparoscopy. Laparoscopic hysterectomy and associated procedures have now become the leading causes of iatrogenic urological injuries.[1] These are notorious for delayed presentation. *Adherence to the safety measures in the use of electrosurgical instruments (monopolar and bipolar), and ultrasonic devices (like harmonic scalpel)* is of paramount importance. Intraoperative identification of ureteric injury is only around 30%. It is therefore imperative that we have a high index of suspicion to identify them.

CARE WHILE OPERATING ON CERVICAL FIBROID AND BROAD LIGAMENT FIBROID

Standard teaching dictates that applying clamps hugging the uterus will prevent ureteric injury. It is not possible to do that if we have a *large cervical fibroid*. The UV fold of the peritoneum (which lies above the junction of the normal-sized body of the uterus and the large cervical fibroid) is opened and the bladder is pushed down. A vertical midline incision can be made on the cervical fibroid slowly, till we reach the pseudo capsule (the plane between the myoma and the cervix). A finger can be insinuated in this relatively avascular plane and the myoma can be enucleated in toto. It is now possible to apply clamps hugging the uterus thereby reducing the threat of ureteric injury **(Fig. 4)**.

In the case of *a broad-ligament fibroid* also, we will not be able to apply clamps close to the uterus. If the leaves of the broad ligament overlying the fibroid are opened, enucleation of the broad-ligament fibroid can be easily achieved. The ureter and iliac vessels can be visualized and safeguarded. We can now proceed with hysterectomy in the usual way without fear of urological injury **(Fig. 5)**.

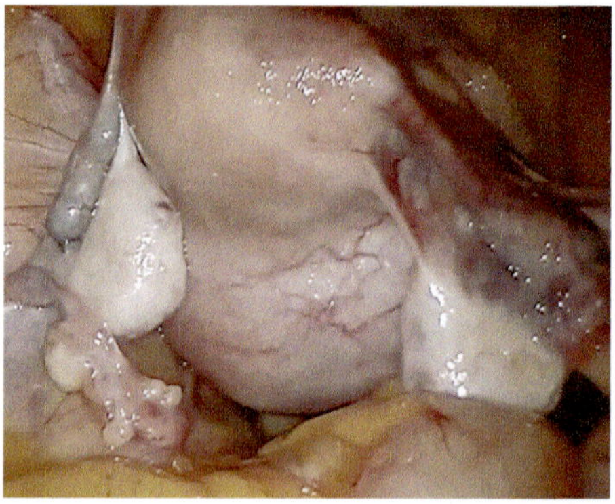

Fig. 4: Cervical fibroid.

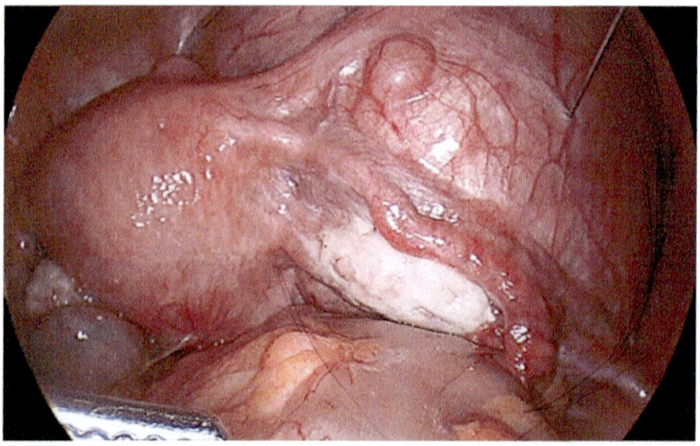

Fig. 5: Broad-ligament fibroid.

Preventive Measures in Severe Adhesions

Careful adhesiolysis must be done in cases where the patient has endometriosis, PID, malignancy, or has undergone multiple surgeries. It is better to ensure that what we are cutting is not the ureter. In case of difficulty or if we have any doubt, it is better to open the retroperitoneum, visualize the ureters and safeguard it.[7]

CARE WHILE PERFORMING APICAL SUSPENSION

Apical suspension plays an important role in the prevention of recurrence. Among the different procedures available, there is a higher incidence of intraoperative injuries with high uterosacral ligament suspension procedures (between 1.8 and 10.9%).[6] We now have different modifications of the procedure which are less risky.[8]

Check cystoscopy will not only assess if there is any ureteric injury, but it will give us an opportunity to rectify them. Sacrospinous ligament fixation and McCall culdoplasty have low rates of ureteral obstruction.[9]

Role of Stenting

Stenting does not always protect against ureteric injury. It is useful for intraoperative recognition and immediate management. Stenting itself rarely can have problems like bleeding, ureteric perforation, edema, and stent malposition. Fibrosis from conditions like endometriosis may make stent palpation and recognition difficult. In case of any doubt, cystoscopy and stenting go a long way in early recognition and management thereby preventing genitourinary fistula.[5]

CARE WHILE OPERATING ON ANTERIOR VAGINAL WALL CYST/SUBURETHRAL CYST

It is better to put an indwelling Foley catheter.

Hydrodissection will help safe reflection of the vaginal walls. While operating on a urethral diverticulum, we will be able to see the Foley catheter, when the cyst wall is removed. The urethra now has to be repaired followed by layered closure **(Fig. 6)**.

Pointers to Bladder Injury

- Identification of a rent in the bladder through which the Foley's catheter is seen.
- Blood-stained urine in the catheter.
- In patients undergoing vaginal hysterectomy, the catheter introduced through the urethra into the bladder can traverse through the rent in the bladder.

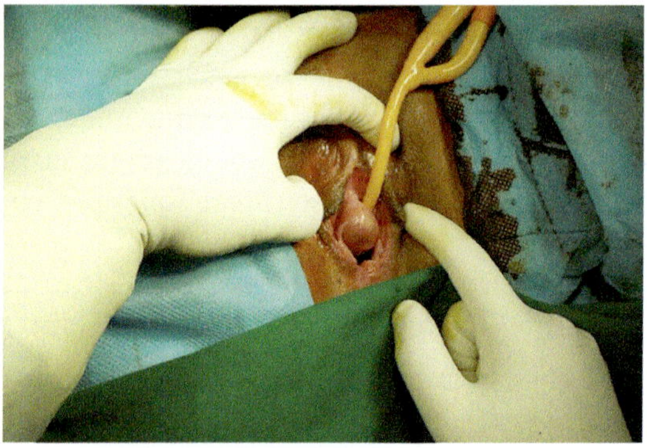

Fig. 6: Anterior vaginal wall cyst/Suburethral cyst.

- Distension of the Urobag with gas occurs in patients undergoing laparoscopic hysterectomy, when there is a bladder injury.
- Methylene blue solution instilled through the urethra into the bladder will come out through the rent in the bladder.
- Cystoscopic confirmation.

What measures should be taken in the event of a suspected ureteric injury?[7,10]

We need to visualize the ureters directly during laparotomy. One cannot rule out ureteric injury because of the presence of ureteric peristalsis. The retroperitoneum can be opened and the ureter visualized completely. Cystoscopy and assessment of ureteric efflux on both sides should be done. In case of any doubt, ureteroscopy and stenting or definite repair according to the situation needs to be done.

PRACTICE POINTS

- Identify patients with risk factors and counsel them adequately with the establishment of preventative strategies.[2]
- Take all steps to avoid any inadvertent injuries.
- Be vigilant enough to recognize any possible injury. A high index of suspicion is needed.
- Provide appropriate remedial measures.
- Patients need to be counseled that despite taking all precautions there is a possibility of inadvertent injury and some of them may have a delayed presentation.

REFERENCES

1. Partin AW, Dmochowski RR, Kavoussi LR, Peters C. Chapter 129. In: Campbell-Walsh-Wein Urology, 12th edn (Vol 3). Philadelphia, PA: Elsevier; 2021. pp. 2924-63.

2. Wei G, Harley F, O'Callaghan M, Adshead J, Hennessey D, Kinnear N. Systematic review of urological injury during cesarean section and hysterectomy. Int Urogynecol J. 2022;34(2):371-89.
3. Tarney C. Bladder injury during cesarean delivery. Current Women's Health Reviews. 2014;9(2):70–6. doi:10.2174/157340480902140102151729
4. Alanwar A, Al-Sayed HM, Ibrahim AM, Elkotb AM, Abdelshafy A, Abdelhadi R, et al. Urinary tract injuries during cesarean section in patients with morbid placental adherence: retrospective cohort study. J Matern Fetal Neonatal Med. 2017;32(9):1461-7.
5. Dallas KB, Rogo-Gupta L, Elliott CS. Urologic injury and fistula after hysterectomy for benign indications. Obstet Gynecol. 2019;134(2):241-9.
6. Smith AP, Bazinet A, Liberman D. Iatrogenic ureteral injury after gynecological surgery. Can Urol Assoc J. 2019; 13(6 Suppl4):S51-S55.
7. Morey A, Broghammer J, Hollowell C, McKibben M, Souter L. UROTRAUMA Guideline 2020: AUA Guideline. J Urol. 2021;205(1):30-5.
8. Pal M. Extraperitoneal high uterosacral ligament suspension. In: Pal M (Ed) Urogynecology & Pelvic Reconstructive Surgery, 2nd edn. New Delhi: Jaypee Brothers Medical Publishers Pvt Ltd; 2024, p 282-287. 10
9. Soma B, Manidip P. Cesarean bladder injury - obstetrician's nightmare. J Family Med Prim Care. 2020;9(9):4526.
10. Nerli R, Ghagane S, Kadeli V, Hiremath M. Ureteric injuries during laparoscopic gynecologic surgeries. J Sci Soc. 2019;46(1):3.

10

CHAPTER

Different Methods of Tissue Dissection in Vaginal Hysterectomy

Sandhya Rani Panigrahy, Partha Sarathi Tripathy

INTRODUCTION

Infiltration of local anesthetics has been used for a very long time in vaginal and perineal surgery. The use of local infiltration which contains adrenaline has been traditionally used to reduce hemorrhage but is known to be associated with tachyarrhythmias when accidentally injected into the vascular system.[1]

A wide variety and concentration of agents are used for local infiltration.

There seems to be no consensus on the type, concentration of agents and concomitant use of vasoconstrictor agents like adrenaline.

There is a paucity of good quality data on outcomes like operation time, analgesia requirements, etc.

When using local infiltration with or without vasoconstrictors our aim is to survey the practice and reasons of use of local infiltration in prolapse and repair surgery.

Surgeons can perform hysterectomy through more than a few different methods. Some of the generally performed routes of hysterectomy are vaginal, abdominal, laparoscopic, and robotic assisted. Vaginal hysterectomy ranks as one of the least and minimally invasive types of hysterectomies, and it has better outcomes and fewer complications compared to other types. It should be regarded as the preferred route of hysterectomy, whenever possible. The advantages of vaginal hysterectomy include less pain, rapid recovery, faster return to work, lower costs, and lower morbidity.[2]

Gynecologists with special interest in urogynecology, urogynecologists, urologists and allied professionals who are doing vaginal surgeries for various indications use infiltration method for hemostasis purpose, Bloodless field and less injury to nearby tissue.

Different Types of Incision

Circumference: Circumferential incision is made around the cervix at the cervicovaginal intersection by using a scalpel or diathermy.

Inverted T: Incision given over the anterior cervicovaginal area to make the uterus free from bladder and give access to anterior entry to abdominal cavity. The free flaps are kept asides from below upwards and at the end of procedure cut and used for tightening of the vaginal.

Inverted V: This is another type of incision given for vaginal hysterectomy over cervicovaginal junction in the anatomical landmark of imaginary triangle of urethra on top and two lateral side broad area of cervicovaginal junction.

L-Longitudinal: Vertical incision given over the cervix on anterior wall top point is suburethral and below cervicovesical junction on vertical way.

DIFFERENT INJECTING AGENTS

- *Injecting vasoconstricting agents:* Dilute vasopressin (20 units in 100 mL of normal saline) is circumferentially injected into the proper planes of the cervicovaginal junction. Maximum 20–30 mL used for this procedure. The purpose of this is for hemostasis and hydrodissection.
- *Hydrodissection:* Injecting normal saline 100–200 mL into the cervicovaginal junction in proper plane.
- The purpose of this procedure is to get into the proper plane of dissection.
- *Injection of adrenaline with normal saline:* An Amp of adrenaline draw, and syringe washed and diluted with 200 mL normal saline, only maximum 20–30 mL solution used. It is a vasoconstrictor agent. With regard to use of adrenaline (90%) used it with local anesthetic.
- The most common concentration of adrenaline used was 1 in 1,000. Though some surgeons diluted it with normal saline to 1 in 100,000. Hemostasis is better and field of operation is more bloodless. It is contraindicated in hypertensive patients and cardiac disease. Tachyarrhythmias is observed in some cases.
- Normal saline in infiltration used by surgeons is 58.7%. The types of local anesthetic used were lignocaine (45.7%), prilocaine with octapressin (13.6%), bupivacine (11.4%), marcaine (9.1%), prilocaine (6.8%), chirocaine (2.3%), and other (10.9%)

DIFFERENT OPERATIVE PROCEDURES

- *Clamping and cutting:* Heaney clamp is widely opened and slide off the cervix, making sure all the vasculature is incorporated into the clamp, uterine vessels are cut, and suture ligated.
- Clampless surgery
- *Sutureless surgery:* Using vessel sealer making the procedure and steps of operations very quick by omitting the clamping and cutting and suturing
- Few surgeons follow the step of suturing the ligaments and cutting them.

- *Bloodless surgery:* Using harmony scalpel and diathermy and vessel sealer is really a boon for vaginal surgeons to make the operation more quick procedure, easy and drop less field during operation.

DIFFERENT TYPES OF TISSUE DISSECTION

- Sharp instrument dissection
- Blunt instrument dissection
- Finger dissection
- Gauze dissection
- Dissection and suturing
- Diathermy cautery dissection and coagulation

For all these operative procedures to follow stepwise as dissection of anterior vaginal wall dissection to open up the abdomen to make free uterus from anterior wall and open up cul-de-sac to free uterus posteriorly.

Sharp dissection is used maintaining the hemostasis by suturing or using diathermy.

Sharp dissection is used when the tissues are tough, tight, fibrosis band are present and large ligaments.

Named vessels should be properly sutured and unknown vessels should be cauterized to make the field of operative procedure bloodless, more visibility and proper hemostasis.

Utero-ovarian, round ligament complex, and cornual end of the Fallopian tube. The upper and the final pedicle can be clamped all together or separately. If the pedicles are too large, the round ligament can be clamped individually. As this is a large pedicle, the author recommends doubly clamping this pedicle, and two sutures are placed. First, suture tie followed by suture ligation medial to the first. Once all ligaments and vessels are cut, ligated, and secured, the uterus is delivered.[3]

Blunt dissection is followed when dealing with more vascular ligaments and large vessels nearby. Hemostasias to maintained to prevent blood loss and speedy recovery.

Gauze dissection followed many years back to get a proper plane in the surgical area and finger or fine artery with gauze followed for this and hemostasis maintained by suturing the bleeding points.

After coming the era of diathermy and harmonic or vessel sealer now a days gauze dissection is outdated.[4]

TOXICITY

- The use of local anesthetics does come with the possibility of side effects.
- The local side effects of most agents are restricted to bruising and temporary sensation of stinging or burning.
- Systemic toxicity manifests as severe numbness, dizziness, tinnitus, slurred speech, seizures, cardiac depression, etc.

- *The toxic effects are usually due to:*
  - Accidental rapid intravenous infusion,
  - Rapid absorption and
  - Excessive use resulting in overdose

This can be avoided with the use of the right technique, concentration and total volume of agent. Care needs to be taken when selecting agents for very old people and for those with significant medical problems, using multiple medications where the possibility of interactions exists.[4]

DISCUSSION

Vaginal hysterectomy is considered one of the minimally invasive forms of hysterectomies with better outcomes and fewer complications.[5] It should be viewed as the preferred mode of hysterectomy whenever possible. The advantages of vaginal hysterectomy include less pain, rapid recovery, faster return to work, lower costs, and lower morbidity. It is usually performed for benign conditions.

While 90% of respondents felt infiltration dissection helps reduce blood loss, only 46% were convinced that it helped reduce visceral injury. The survey reflects that the majority surgeons use local infiltration for gynecological surgery.

FOR BEST OUTCOME

- The only way to achieve the best outcome in patients undergoing vaginal hysterectomy and their families is through coordinated care among the interprofessional team members.
- Time out (pre-procedure verification checklist) is always performed before the commencement of surgery to confirm the correct patient, type of the operation, equipment used, and the surgeon performing the procedure, as per the standard hospital protocol.
- The patient is examined under anesthesia for the evaluation of size, shape, mobility of the uterus, assessment of the adnexa, and other pelvic structures. The degree of descent of the uterus, vaginal wall caliber, and pelvic organ prolapse, cystocele, and rectocele are assessed.[6]
- Never do operation on a time basis, it is always case basis.
- Never compare with other colleagues compete with yourself.
- Never compromise with instruments, sutures and bleeding points.
- Never be afraid to change over to the abdominal route when there is any complications or difficulties in operation by vaginal route.
- The survey was designed with the intention of identifying variation in current practice for use of local infiltration, and perception of practitioners about its advantages. A response rate of 51% was achieved. The survey

reflects that the majority use local infiltration for gynecological surgery; however, there is wide variation in the type and strengths of agents used.

- Use of vasoconstrictors is common practice as well, but there was variation in the strength used. Whilst 90% respondents felt it helped reduce blood loss, only 46% were convinced that it helped reduce visceral injury. There is some literature to suggest that hydrodissection does not reduce the risk of visceral injury. Almost half of the respondents (46%) felt that it provided some pain relief.
- Gynecological surgery is moving more and more towards daycare surgery, as it is financially much more viable and also associated with significantly less side effects when compared to surgery under general anesthetic or spinal anesthetic.
- It would also be a choice where a general anesthetic or spinal anesthetic is contraindicated because of medical conditions like asthma, cardiac disease, spinal problems, etc.
- Though the majority of respondents felt that local infiltration provided better planes of dissection, there is no evidence to support this opinion in vaginal or other surgery.
- Side effects emanating from the usage of local anesthetic can be reduced by the use of vasoconstrictors, which reduces the speed of absorption by as much as 50%.
- Adrenaline, however, has side effects such as tachyarrhythmias.
- There is evidence to support local anesthetic use to reduce postoperative analgesic requirements.
- There is some evidence to suggest the same in pelvic floor surgery, but the data are not very robust.
- Earlier studies showed a 58% reduction in blood loss and reduction of blood transfusion from four-fifths to one-third, whilst another study showed an appreciable reduction in blood loss (27.7%) when epinephrine (1:200,000) was used for local infiltration in vaginal hysterectomy.
- A study comparing the reduction in blood loss using two strengths of adrenaline versus no adrenaline of vaginal surgery concluded that adrenaline in strengths of 1:120,000 and 1:240,000 showed a significant reduction in blood loss.
- There might be differences in outcomes like blood loss depending on the type of vasoconstrictor used.
- However, there have been questions raised regarding the increased risk of infection with impairment of tissue defenses by vasoconstrictors in vaginal hysterectomies.
- There is wide variation in the use of local anesthetic and vasoconstrictors in pelvic floor surgery. There is a need for a robustly designed randomized controlled trial for use of local anesthetic with and without vasoconstrictors in pelvic floor surgery to study outcomes like reduction in

visceral injuries, reduction in operation time and postoperative analgesia requirements, as well as adverse events like tachyarrhythmias and infections.

REFERENCES

1. Dedden SJ, Geomini PMAJ, Huirne JAF, Bongers MY. Vaginal and laparoscopic hysterectomy as an outpatient procedure: a systematic review. Eur J Obstet Gynecol Reprod Biol. 2017;216:212-23. [PubMed]
2. ACOG Practice Bulletin No 195. Prevention of infection after gynecologic procedures. Obstet Gynecol. 2018;131(6):e172-89. [PubMed]
3. Humes JC, Weir L, Keyser EA, Molina MM. The dying art of vaginal hysterectomy: a novel simulation. Cureus. 2019;11(12):e6362. [PMC free article] [PubMed]
4. Latthe P, Kadian S, Parsons M, Toozs-Hobson P. Survey of use of local infiltration and vasoconstrictors in vaginal surgery. Gynecol Surg. 2007;4(3):187-9.
5. O'Neal MG, Beste T, Shackelford DP. Utility of preemptive local analgesia in vaginal hysterectomy. Am J Obstet Gynecol. 2003;189(6):1539.
6. Ghezzi F, Cromi A, Raio L, Bergamini V, Triacca P, Serati M, et al. Influence of the type of anesthesia and hydrodissection on the complication rate after tension-free vaginal tape procedure. Eur J Obstet Gynecol Reprod Biol. 2005;118(1):96-100.

11

CHAPTER

Perineal Tears

Samir R Pradhan

INTRODUCTION

Perineal tears can occur during a vaginal delivery either spontaneously or following an extension of episiotomy (a surgical incision of the perineum).

There are four degrees of perineal tears[1] **(Fig. 1)**:

1. *First degree:* Least severe, involves only the first layer of skin.
2. *Second degree:* Involves skin and underlying muscles of perineum.
3. *Third degree:* Involves disruption of anal sphincter muscles.
   a. Partial disruption (less than 50%) of external anal sphincter.
   b. Total disruption (more than 50%) of external anal sphincter.
   c. Disruption of external and internal anal sphincter.

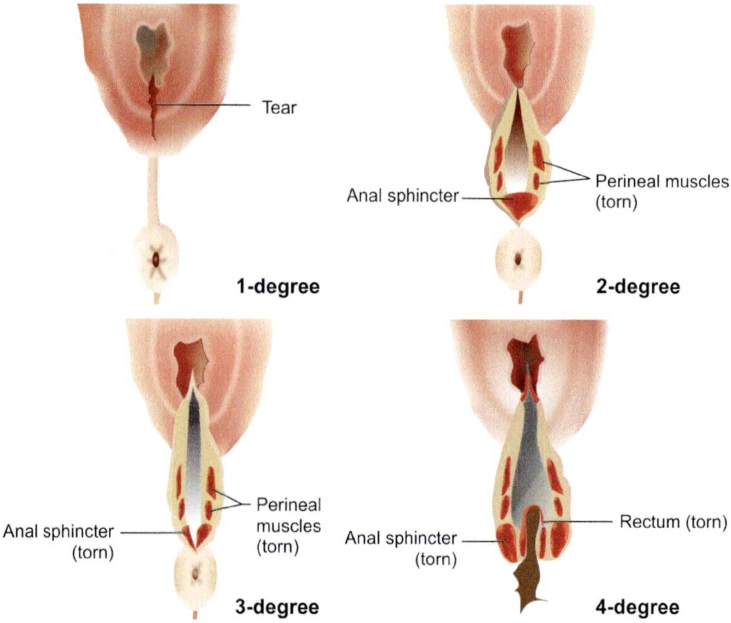

Fig. 1: Manual on Vaginal Surgery AICOG 2013 Mumbai.

4. *Fourth degree:* Involves breach in anal mucosa in addition to third degree.

Obstetric anal sphincter injury (OASI) encompasses third degree and fourth degree perineal tears. These are important cause of anal dysfunction in women. They have a severe impact on quality-of-life.

Rectal buttonhole injury: Tear involves the rectal mucosa with an intact anal sphincter.

Undiagnosed or suboptimal OASI repair can cause:

- Fecal incontinence
- Flatus incontinence
- Significant deterioration of quality-of-life
- Abscess formation
- Wound breakdown
- Rectovaginal fistula
- Old complete perineal tear
- Risk of litigation

INCIDENCE

The overall incidence in the UK is 2.9% (primigravida 6.1%; multigravida 1.7%).[2] The prevalence of OASI in the general population is between 0.5 to 5%. A higher prevalence of 1 to 15% is reported in the case of operative vaginal delivery.

RISK FACTORS[3]

A. *Maternal:*
   a. Primipara
   b. Asian ethnicity[4]

B. *Intrapartum:*
   a. Induction of labor
   b. Epidural analgesia
   c. Instrumental delivery, especially Forceps
   d. Prolonged second stage of labor
   e. Shoulder dystocia
   f. Midline episiotomy

C. *Fetal:*
   a. Weight over 4 kg
   b. Persistent occipito-posterior position
   c. Postmaturity

DIAGNOSIS

- Increased vigilance about OASI
- Counsel regarding need for vaginal and rectal examination after delivery

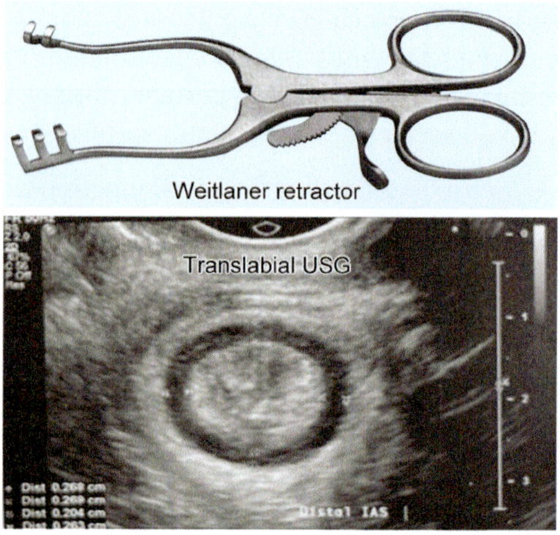

Fig. 2: Manual of Vaginal Surgery and Urogynecology, AICOG 2020, Lucknow.

- Good lighting
- Lithotomy position
- Visual inspection of perineum and vagina including identification of Apex
- Per-rectal examination
- Digital palpation. Examiner's dominant index finger in the anus and ipsilateral thumb on the perineum at 9 o'clock and pill rolling motion from 9 o'clock to 3 o'clock
- External anal sphincter appears like red meat.
- Internal anal sphincter appears pale like Salmon fish and is 6 mm to 8 mm cephalad to the anal margin.
- Weitlander retractor can be used **(Fig. 2)**.
- Translabial ultrasound if facilities and expertise are available **(Fig. 2)**.

PREVENTION OF PERINEAL TRAUMA

A. *Antenatal:*[5]
   - Perineal massage performed during last 4–6 weeks of pregnancy daily for 10 minutes.
   - Increases elasticity of perineum and relaxes muscles of perineal area.

   Technique: Wash hands, lubricate thumbs and perineal tissues, place thumbs 1 inch inside vagina, press down and to the sides as shown in **Figure 3**, hold position for 1–2 minutes, then with thumbs, massage using U-shaped movement.

B. *Intranatal* ***(Fig. 3)****:*
   a. *Perineal massage:*[6] Two fingers of the nurse's gloved hand to be moved side to side inside the patient's vagina with mild gentle downward

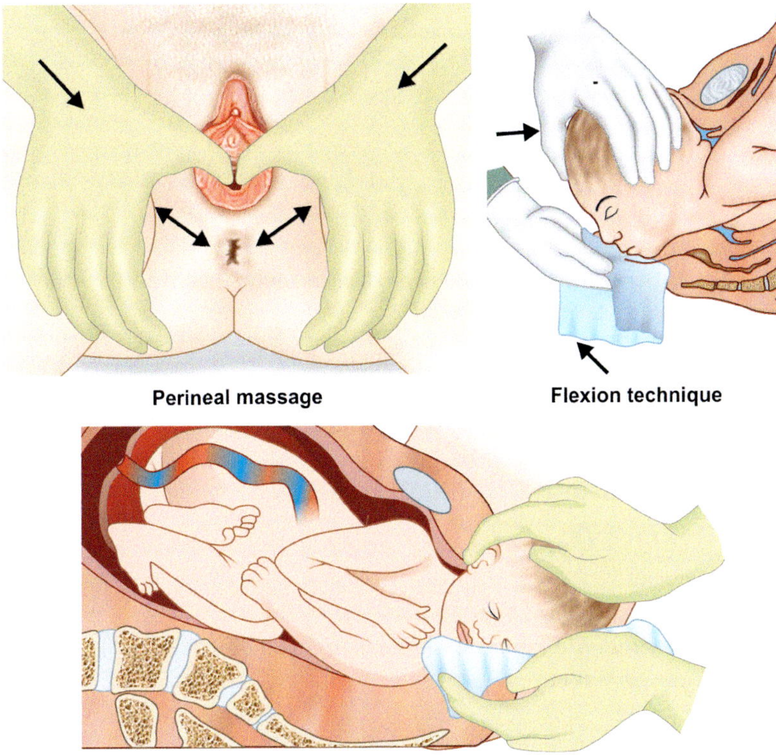

Fig. 3: FOGSI Recent advances—Perineal Disorders.

steady pressure towards rectum. Massage to be used between the pushes during second stage.

b. *Warm towels*[6] *(Albers 2005):* Used at mother's perineum in first stage.

c. *Flexion technique (De Wees, 1889):* Maintain the flexion of emerging head by pressing the emerging occiput in a downwards direction towards the perineum and preventing its extension until crowning.

d. *Ritgen's maneuver (Williams' Obstetrics, 1st edition, 1903):* Performed between contraction wherein the fetal chin is reached between the anus and coccyx and pulled inferiorly while fingers of the other hand on the fetal occiput control the speed of delivery.

e. *Finnish maneuver:*[7] Speed of crowning is controlled by exerting pressure on occiput with one hand. Simultaneously, the thumb and index finger of the other hand are used to support the perineum while the flexed middle finger takes a grip of the baby's chin. Subsequently, the parturient stops pushing, breathes rapidly and the accoucheur slowly helps the baby's head through the introitus. When most of the head is out, the perineal ring is pushed under the baby's chin **(Fig. 4)**.

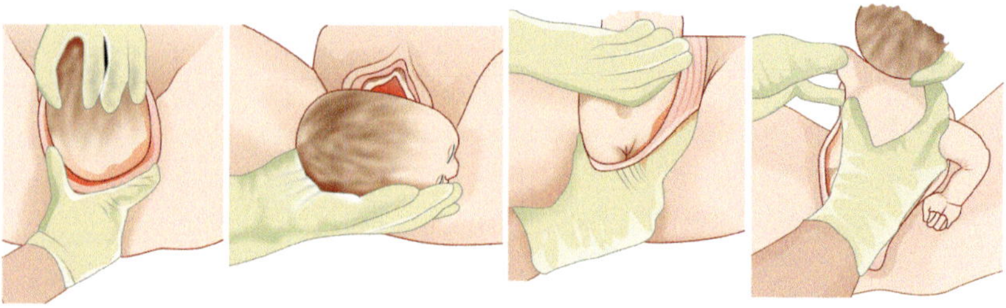

Fig. 4: (Hana Kleprlikova—youtube video:Maternity & Midwifery Forum)

f. Mediolateral episiotomy at an angle of 60° from center of introitus at crowning,[8] especially for operative vaginal delivery.
The resultant postdelivery angle is 45°.

PRIMARY REPAIR OF PERINEAL TEAR[9]

General Principles

- Real consent
- Aseptic precautions in operation theater
- *Adequate suitable anesthesia:* General, regional or local (1°, 2°)
- Adequate assistance
- Good lighting
- Appropriate instruments (Weitlaner retractor)
- Lithotomy position
- *Suture materials:*
  - *Anal mucosa:* 3-0 Polyglactin (Vicryl)
  - *Internal and external anal sphincter:* 3-0 Polydioxanone (PDS) or 2-0 Polyglactin
  - *Perineal muscles, vaginal mucosa, Skin:* 2-0 Polyglactin (Vicryl) or Vicryl Rapide

First degree tear needs repair only if there is excess bleeding or raw surface exposure is more. It is done under LA with interrupted sutures approximating the torn mucosal edge.

Second degree tear mimics midline episiotomy. Apex visualization is important. Vaginal mucosa with rectovaginal fascia is sutured in continuous interlocking suture. Transverse perineal muscles are approximated in interrupted sutures. Skin repaired with simple sutures, vertical mattress sutures or subcuticular sutures.

Third degree and fourth degree tear (OASI): To be done by trained personnel

- *Anal mucosa:* Continuous or interrupted. Knots outside anal lumen
- *Internal anal sphincter (IAS):* It plays an important role in the maintenance of continence. IAS contributes to the bulk of anal canal resting pressure.

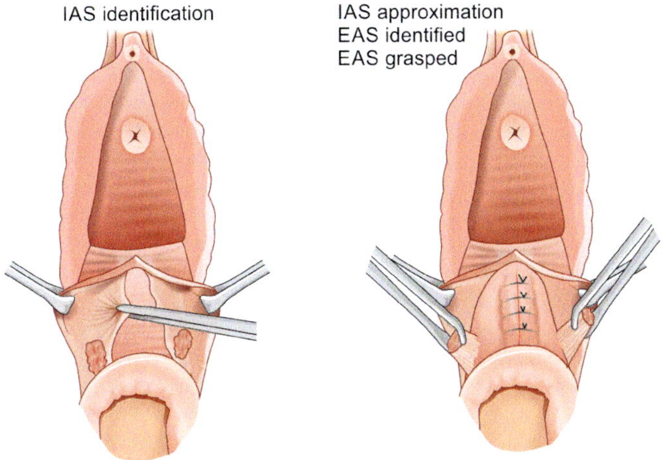

Fig. 5: Anal mucosa. (EAS: external anal sphincter; IAS: internal anal sphincter)
Source: Williams Gynecology, 2nd edition, pg. 1253.

It has to be identified and sutured separately with horizontal mattress (end-to-end sutures) without overlap.

- *External anal sphincter (EAS):* It maintains constant resting contraction to aid continence and provides an additional squeeze when continence is threatened. EAS is under tonic contraction, so when torn its ends retract and the repair involves identification and grasping of the torn ends using Allis tissue forceps **(Fig. 5)**.
- Mobilization from ischioanal fat required using fine scissors especially if overlap planned.
- Avoid Figure-of-8 sutures as they can cause ischemia.
- PR required after repair to ensure that anal mucosa is not inadvertently included.
- *If partial thickness (3a and some 3b):* Technique is End to End.
- *If complete thickness (3b):* Technique is overlap[10] or end to end. Both have equal outcomes.[11] However, the overlap technique gives better apposition, longer anal length, greater surface area of contact and better muscle continuity **(Fig. 6)**.

POST-REPAIR MANAGEMENT[9]

- Foley's catheterization of urinary bladder for 24 hours to avoid urinary retention due to severe perineal discomfort or regional anesthesia.
- Broad-spectrum antibiotics cephalosporins and metronidazole parenteral followed by oral for 5 days to avoid wound breakdown due to infection.
- No need of excess starvation. Low residue diet with adequate hydration.
- Laxatives like lactulose are preferable for 10 days post-repair.
- Avoid constipating agents or bulk laxatives.[12]

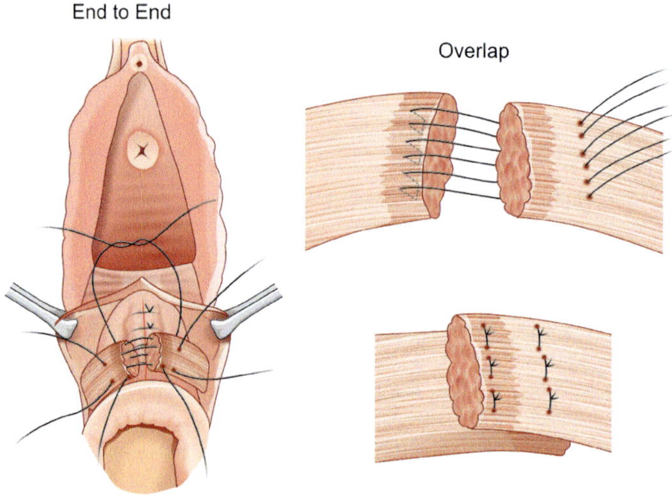

Fig. 6: Repair of external anal sphincter.

- Analgesics like diclofenac (suppository) for 48 hours.
- Use of warm sitz bath, donut-shaped pillow.
- Avoid exercises that aggravate perineal area like squatting or walking down steps.
- Early physiotherapy and pelvic floor exercises for 6–12 weeks.
- Review by treating obstetrician after 6–12 weeks.
- If pain or fecal incontinence or flatus incontinence, endoanal ultrasound, anorectal manometry and referral to colorectal surgeon.
- Risk of recurrence in subsequent delivery is 5–7%, and to be counseled about risk of developing anal incontinence or worsening symptoms with subsequent delivery and should be given an option of elective cesarean birth.

REFERENCES

1. Sultan AH. Obstetric perineal injury and anal incontinence. Clin Risk. 1999;5:193-6.
2. Thiagamoorthy G, Johnson A, Thakar R, Sultan AH. National Survey of Perineal Trauma and its Subsequent Management in the United Kingdom. Int Urogynecol J Pelvic Floor Dysfunction. 2014;25(12):1621-7.
3. Riskin-Mashiash S, Wilkins IA, et al. Risk factors for severe perineal tear: can we do better? Am J Perinatol. 2002;19:225-34.
4. Goldberg J, Hyslop T, et al. Racial differences in severe perineal lacerations after vaginal delivery. Am J Obstet Gynecol. 2003;188:1063-7.
5. Beckmann MM, Stock OM. Antenatal perineal massage for reducing perineal trauma. Cochrane Database Syst Rev. 2013;(4):CD005123.

6. Aasheim V, Nilsen AB, Lukasse M, et al. Perineal techniques during the second stage of labour for reducing perineal trauma. Cochrane Database Syst Rev. 2011;(12):CD006672.
7. Poulsen MO, Madsen ML, et al. Does the Finnish intervention prevent OASI? A systematic review of literature. BMJ Open. 2015;5(9):8346.
8. Okeahialam N, Wong KW, Jha S, Sultan AH, Thakar R. Mediolateral episiotomy with operative vaginal delivery and the risk reduction of OASI: a systematic review and meta-analysis. Int Urogynecol J. 2022:33(6):1393-405.
9. Royal College of Obstetricians and Gynaecologists (RCOG). The Management of Third and Fourth Degree Perineal Tears. RCOG Green-top guideline No 29. June 2015.
10. Parks AG. Royal Society of Medicine, Section of Proctology: Meeting 27 November 1974. President"s Address. Anorectal Incontinence. Proc R Soc Med. 1975;68(11).681-90.
11. Fernando RJ, Sultan AH, et al. Methods of repair for OASI. Cochrane Database Syst Rev. 2006;(3):CD002866.
12. Eogan M, Daly L, Behan M, et al. Randomized clinical trial of bowel confinement vs laxative use after primary repair of OASI. BJOG. 2007:114:736-40.

12 CHAPTER

Vault Prolapse

Rajendra Saraogi, Sonam Kataria

DEFINITION

Descent of the vault below a point 2 cm less than the total vaginal length above the plane of hymen.[1]

INTRODUCTION

Vault prolapse is the herniation of the pelvic organs to or beyond the vaginal walls. It is reported to be the most common reason for hysterectomy in elderly.

INCIDENCE

The overall incidence of prolapse is 2–43%. Hysterectomies performed for prolapse is 11.6% and 1.8% is for other benign diseases. It can also occur months-years after the hysterectomy with other pelvic floor defects such as cystocele, rectocele, and enterocele. The number of women with pelvic organ prolapse who are managed without hospitalization and surgery and the number of women with prolapse who never seek medical treatment are unknown.

ANATOMY—VAGINAL VAULT SUPPORT

Maintenance of normal vaginal anatomy depends on the inter-relationships of intact pelvic floor neuromuscular ligaments and fascia. This complex relationship of vaginal support is perhaps least understood at the vaginal apex or vault. Without proper identification and correction of vaginal vault prolapse, surgical correction of the other vaginal compartments is likely to fail. This contributes to the 29.2% re-operation rate of women who undergo pelvic floor reconstruction. In a nonhysterectomized women, the vault or apex is located posterior and superior to the cervix. After hysterectomy, the scar site assumes the position of the vaginal apex or vault.

RELEVANT ANATOMY

The vaginal apex is a site at which multiple vaginal support structures converge. If the cervix is present, it serves as a strong attachment point for the ligaments and fascia. A woman who has had a prior hysterectomy may not have a strong attachment point leading to vault support weakness and potential prolapse.

Delancey's Three-level Connective Tissue Support of the Vagina

Level I support is composed of the uterosacral/cardinal ligament complex that originates at the cervix and upper vagina and inserts at the pelvic sidewall and sacrum. This ligamentous complex suspends at the uterus and upper vagina in its normal orientation. It helps maintain vaginal length and normal vaginal axis. The loss of level I support contributes to prolapse of the vaginal apex.

Level II support comprises the paravaginal attachments of full length of the vagina and are suspended by the arcus tendinous fascia pelvis (ATFP) or lateral pelvic white line. Loss of level II support contributes to cystocele (anterior vaginal prolapse).

Level III support is provided by the perineal membrane, perineal body, superficial and deep perineal muscles. As stated above, it is the level I support the uterosacral/cardinal ligament complex that plays the most important role in maintaining vaginal vault support. The endopelvic fascia is the fibromuscular tissue that underlies the vaginal epithelium. This layer envelopes the entire vaginal canal extending from apex to perineum and arcus tendinous to arcus tendinous.

VAULT PROLAPSE

This occurs due to deficiency in anterior compartment, middle compartment, posterior compartment. This can occur with an intact uterus or after removal of uterus. The incidence of vault prolapse following hysterectomy by any route practically remains the same.

POP-Q classification demonstration of vault prolapse is shown in **Figure 1**.

Preventable and Nonpreventable Factors for Vault Prolapse

Nonpreventable factors for vault prolapse are aging, ethnicity and racial factors, connective tissue disorders, neurologic disorders, menopause due to estrogen deficiency.

Preventable factors are obstetric factors like forceps assisted vaginal delivery, prolonged second stage of labor causing nerve and muscular damage of the pelvic floor, obesity increased intra-abdominal pressure—constipation, multiparity hysterectomy: vault prolapse can occur if proper care is not taken to support the vaginal vault and obliterate the cul-de-sac, by McCall culdoplasty at the time of VH reduces PHVP.

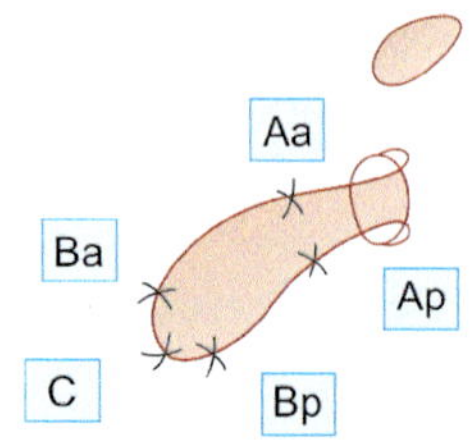

+2 Aa	+7 Ba	+7 C
5 gh	1 pb	7 tvl
+2 Ap	+7 Bp	– D

Fig. 1: POP-Q classification demonstration of vault prolapse.

Similarly, suturing cardinal and uterosacral ligaments to vaginal cuff at the time of vaginal and abdominal hysterectomy.

Sacrospinous fixation to be considered at the time of vaginal hysterectomy in case of descent of vaginal cuff up to introitus. Avoid subtotal hysterectomy. Uterosacral ligament suspension may be performed at the time of abdominal and laparoscopic hysterectomy. Sacrospinous ligament fixation and abdominal sacrocolpopexy are not recommended for the prevention of prolapse at the time of hysterectomy done for no prolapse-related diseases.

TREATMENT

Palliative Treatment

If you do not treat, only 20% will get worse. Lifestyle changes by losing weight which will decrease the BMI, avoiding smoking and treating chronic cough.

Palliative treatment like silicone pessary is useful in very old frail patients, medically unfit patients. Patient not willing for the surgery Kegel's exercise is useful in mild symptomatic patients. It increases the tone of pelvic floor muscles and prevents the progression of the disease. Other palliative treatment like electric muscle stimulation, perineometer, vaginal cone, etc., can be tried.

Surgical Treatment

Principles of Reconstructive Surgeries

"The type of the operation performed should be tailored to the individual case."

Discuss with the patient various routes and options with pros and cons. Consider patient's age, co-morbid conditions and pathology if any, avoid distortion of vaginal axis, preserve adequate vaginal length (≥7) as well as normal vaginal caliber. correct all defects. Choose appropriate surgery for the patient.

Vaginal procedures like sacrospinous fixation, McCall culdoplasty, Iliococcygeus fixation, uterosacral suspension, posterior intravaginal slingplasty.

Obliterative procedures like LeFort's Colpocleisis—complete or partial Goodall power modification, Dani stitch.

Transvaginal mesh:

Trocar-based vaginal kits procedures like Prolift, Apogee, Perigee, and Avulta.

Nontrocar guided—Elevata, Pinnacle, and Uphold

Abdominal procedures like laparotomy/laparoscopy, colposacropexy, high uterosacral ligament suspension, Williams-Richardson operation.

Master et al. (ACOG, 2004) compared both abdominal as well as vaginal procedures by randomized prospective studies and concluded that both the procedures are equally effective on long-term follow-up.

Sacrospinous fixation is better if posterior wall prolapse is predominant.

Abdominal sacropexy is better when anterior vaginal wall is predominant.

Use of mesh vaginally is not recommended to prevent prolapse of vault prolapse. Mesh causes erosion infection, dyspareunia in many cases. FDA has put mesh in category 3 (high-risk category for treatment of prolapse).

VAGINAL PROCEDURES

McCall Culdoplasty

It was introduced by McCall in 1957.[2] It involves plication of the uterosacral ligaments in the midline while reefing the cul-de-sac peritoneum, including full thickness of the apical vaginal mucosa, in a posterior culdoplasty. It is typically done at the time of vaginal hysterectomy and uses nonabsorbable sutures although delayed absorbable sutures may be used. As a general rule, the authority tries to place the uppermost suture on the uterosacral ligaments at a distance from the cuff equal to the amount of vault prolapse present.

Webb et al. followed patients up to 8.8 years and reported 71% did not require any further prolapse operation. They also found 82% were very satisfied or somewhat satisfied with their results.

Uterosacral Ligament Suspension

Reattaching the uterosacral ligaments to the vaginal apex is likely the most physiologic approach to vault prolapse. The technique involves opening the vaginal wall over the apical defect into the peritoneal cavity and identifying the pubocervical fascia, rectovaginal fascia, and uterosacral ligaments.

A permanent 1-0 suture as well as one delayed absorbable 1-0 suture is placed in the posteromedial aspect to each ischial spine. Next, one arm of the permanent and the delayed absorbable suture are placed through pubocervical and rectovaginal fascia as well as the vaginal epithelium at the apex. After any additional vaginal repairs are completed, the sutures are tied elevating the vaginal vault. If extensive vaginal prolapse exists redundant peritoneal tissues can sometimes make identifying the uterosacral ligaments difficult. The ureters lay approximately 1-2 cm lateral to the uterosacral ligaments at the level of the cervix, so being cautious to not kink or injure the ureters when placing the sutures is important. Cystoscopy with visualization of ureteral patency usually with administration of intravenous indigo carmine is recommended following the procedure. Success rates for uterosacral ligament suspension are 87-90% but ureteral injury has been reported to be as high as 11% making it a limiting factor in the success of the technique. Given this reported high complication rate, cystoscopy following suspension is essential.

Iliococcygeus Suspension

This technique involves elevating the apex to the iliococcygeus muscle overlying fascia along the lateral pelvic sidewall. It is a safe and simple procedure and can be done without any vaginal incision by pacing a monofilament permanent suture into the muscle through the vaginal wall either unilaterally or bilaterally. It can be used when isolated unilateral vaginal vault prolapse occurs which can develop following a unilateral sacrospinous fixation or because of a high unilateral paravaginal defect. The presence of permanent suture at the vaginal apex can potentially cause dyspareunia so this technique should be used with caution in women who are sexually active. It is the most useful as a salvage procedure for unilateral apical prolapse. The suspension can also be performed at the time of a posterior wall dissection in which the sutures are placed into the fascia overlying the iliococcygeus, anterior to the ischial spine along the arcus tendinous fascia pelvis and incorporating the pubocervical fascia anteriorly and the rectovaginal fascia posteriorly.

Shull et al. reported 95% cure rate of vault prolapse following iliococcygeus suspension however he also found 14 % rate of prolapse at other sites during the follow-up period. A randomized controlled trial comparing iliococcygeus suspension with sacrospinous fixation demonstrated similar outcomes.

Suspension of the vaginal apex to the sacrospinous ligaments is one of the most commonly performed vault suspensions. It can be performed unilaterally or bilaterally but bilateral fixation avoids vaginal axis deviation giving a more physiological correction of the vaginal vault prolapse. Sacrospinous fixation is performed by entering the pararectal space through a posterior wall dissection. The sacrospinous ligaments are identified running from the ischial spine to the sacrum. Next, 2 nonabsorbable sutures are placed through the ligament not around it as the pudendal nerve and the vessels sit right behind the ligament and damage to these structures can cause significant morbidity. The first suture is placed 2 cm medial to the ischial spine and the second 1 cm medial to the first. Each suture is then passed through the vaginal apex so that when tied the apex is reapproximated to the ligament. Any additional reconstructive procedures are then performed. The success rate of sacrospinous fixation is greater than 90% in multiple series. The concern lies in the exaggerated horizontal axis in which the procedure leaves the vagina, which increases force on the anterior compartment with increases in abdominal pressure. This is especially true if an anti-incontinence procedure is performed at the same time. The rate of cystocele formation following sacrospinous fixation is reported at 20–30% other complications of the procedure include hemorrhage, vaginal shortening, sexual dysfunction and buttock pain.

Advantages

Extraperitoneal, not difficult to perform, low postoperative morbidity, associated anterior and posterior vaginal wall repairs can be done.

Disadvantages

High failure rate compared with abdominal sacrocolpopexy, difficult to perform in short vagina, unilateral vaginal deflection, occasionally nerve injuries and vessel injuries, should not be considered in pre-existing dyspareunia.

LeFort's Colpocleisis

- It is recommended when coital function is not required.
- Quadrilateral flaps from anterior and posterior vaginal walls are removed and raw areas are sutured together.

There are up to 30% chances of postoperative stress urinary incontinence (SUI).

Advantages

- It can be performed under local anesthesia or xylocard.
- It is very simple.
- It can be performed rapidly.
- It gives good satisfactory results.
- It can be performed with 3rd degree uterine descent with cystocele rectocele.
- It can be performed in cases of procidentia.
- It can be performed in vault prolapse repair.

Contraindications: Patient with intact uterus who is not menopause, bad cervix, uterine pathology, patient desires of sexual function.

Disadvantages

It can result in SUI, hematoma.

TECHNIQUE OF OPERATION

Original LeFort operation included making raw surfaces 4 cm in length and 2 cm in breadth on both anterior and posterior vaginal walls.

The raw areas were joined beginning with ends close to the cervix. The reduction progresses step by step with placing of the sutures and when two surfaces are united throughout reduction to complete. Ancillary surgery which can be performed with this is additional perineorrhaphy which can give good support to the perineum.

SUI surgery in the form of Kelly's stitch, meshplasty, TVT, TOT can be performed.

Goodall–Power's Modification of LeFort Operation (1937)

It can be performed in patients with intact nonpathological uterus. A triangular area of vagina is marked about 2 cm above the cervix, the apex of the triangle covering about 1/3 of the length of the vagina sufficient space is left laterally to allow for drainage for cervical secretions. This area of vagina is denuded of mucosa. The same step is repeated on the posterior wall mucosal edges of triangle basis are approximated with 1-0 vicryl. Further closure of the denuded area is done as Le Fort operation. Thus, the obliterated vagina forms a kind of shelf on which the cervix rests with satisfactory drainage of cervical secretions. The resultant vagina is short is functionally satisfactory. Patients with cystocele and rectocele require repairs in the usual way. The cystocele repair is done before tying the lateral surface placed over the denuded area.

Advantages

Vagina is functioning satisfactory—1/3 length of vagina is preserved and sexual function is well.

Disadvantages

Cystocele and rectocele are to be repaired separately.

Dani Stitch

Dr Suhas Dani from Government Medical College performed this operation for the first time. It was published in JOGI in 1989. It is called introital tightening like Thiersch's stitch for rectal prolapse using Sutupak.

Advantages

Less tissue trauma, decrease bleeding, no SUI pap smear can be taken free drainage of vaginal secretion.

The importance of sexual function should be assessed. If the patient has vaginal sexual dysfunction, then sacrocolpopexy should be the primary consideration, given it will avoid any vaginal incisions and potentially avoid vaginal shortening or narrowing. The examiner should assess vaginal length. A woman whose apex reaches the ischial spines without difficulty will likely be successful with a vaginal procedure. If the apex does not reach the spines or reaches well beyond them, she may be better served with either an obliterative procedure or abdominal colpopexy.

TRANSVAGINAL MESH KITS

Vaginal mesh kits can be divided into trocar-based kits that use a transobturator or transgluteal approach to suspend the vagina and nontrocar kits that use a transvaginal fixation method. The trocar-guided kits include Prolift, Apogee and Perigee and Avulta. Trocar-guided kits use a precut sheet of graft material with arms that are used for fixation. Nontrocar kits include Elevate and Pinnacle and Uphold.

With either type of kit some basic surgical principles apply: the vagina should be well estrogenized before the surgery and any vaginal pessary should be removed for 2 weeks prior to surgery to avoid any vaginal epithelium irritation. Exposure of the correct vesicovaginal and rectovaginal planes can be accomplished through hydrodissection, lidocaine with epinephrine, dilute pitressin, or normal saline can be used. Correct hydro-dissection should create a bubble in the avascular space. Mesh should be placed loosely because it can contract upto 20% after placement which can compromise vaginal length and caliber. On July 13th, 2011, the FDA issued a statement that serious complications are very common with the use of surgical mesh in transvaginal repair of pelvic organ prolapse. They also found that mesh in the transvaginal repair of pelvic organ prolapse does not improve symptoms or quality of life. The review found that most common complication was erosion of the mesh through the vagina which can take multiple surgeries to repair and can be debilitating in some women. Mesh contraction was also reported which causes vaginal shortening, tightening and pain.

Apogee Vaginal Vault Suspension

The Apogee system creates neo-ligaments that are analogous to the cardinal by anchoring graft arms at the sites adjacent to the ischial spines, at the attachment of the arcus tendinous.

The technique is performed by accessing the pararectal space and palpating the ischial spine and arcus tendinous. A modified SPARC needle is passed through a pararectal incision that is made 3 cm lateral and 3 cm posterior to the anus. The needle is then guided through the ipsilateral levators and then through the iliococcygeus muscle ultimately anchoring into the arcus tendinous at the level of the ischial spine. The exact anchoring point for the apogee is 0.5–1 cm anterior to the ischial spine through the white line. The polypropylene mesh arms are attached to the needle and brought through the para-anal incision. The graft is secured to the vaginal apex and the perineal body by interrupted delayed absorbable sutures. This recreates apical support from the ischial spine to ischial spine and gives physiologic vaginal axis. Vaginal length averages 7–9 cm and success rate is 88–100% with minimal complications. It is available in synthetic polypropylene mesh and biologic porcine dermis.

Prolift

The Prolift system uses a slightly curved C-shaped trocar to anchor either into the arcus tendinous fascia pelvis (ATFP) or the sacrospinous ligament depending on the approach taken. The graft material is then laid down in a tension-free fashion.

Elmer et al. found that the anatomic cure rate at one year for anterior repair was 79% while 82% for posterior repair and for combined anterior and posterior repair cure rate was 81%. They also found that mesh erosions occurred in 11% of the cases.

Avulta

The Avulta system is another trocar based vaginal mesh kit. It is similar to the above-mentioned kits as trocars are used to fixate synthetic mesh. Dissection is also similar and is done up to the level of the ischial spines. The anterior kit fixation point is 1–2 cm lateral and 3 cm posterior to the ATFP near the ischial spine. The posterior fixation point is the sacrospinous ligament at the ischial spine. The Avulta comes as a posterior or an anterior kit. The posterior kit addresses both the vaginal vault and the posterior vaginal compartment while the anterior kit is used to treat cystoceles.

Elevate

The elevate apical prolapse repair system is a single incision procedure that uses small polypropylene fixation anchors to affix polypropylene mesh arms to the sacrospinous ligaments. The advantage is that the anchors are able to access the sacrospinous ligament without going through or behind it avoiding potential neurovascular complications. The procedure is started with a midline vaginal incision along the anterior or posterior vaginal walls, which is used to access the sacrospinous ligaments and ischial spine through the paravaginal space.

NONTROCAR KITS

Pinnacle and Uphold

The advantage of nontrocar kits is the complete vaginal approach. These kits avoid the transobturator space so surgeons who are not familiar or comfortable with the area can still use a vaginal mesh kit for suspension of the vagina with a total vaginal approach, no blind procedures exist the mesh appendage placement can be done under direct visualization.

Abdominal Procedures

Abdominal Sacral Colpopexy

This is considered by most surgeons to be the criterion standard procedure for repair of vaginal vault prolapse. Although the procedure requires an abdominal incision and has a higher overall morbidity compared to vaginal procedures its longevity and physiologic results as well as having the least risk of sexual dysfunction and dyspareunia make it very appealing.

The procedure begins through an abdominal incision then exposing the sacral promontory by incising the peritoneum between the right ureter and the sigmoid colon. Sutures 2-0 polypropylene or bone anchors are used to place 2-3 sacral suspensory sutures. Next the vaginal apex is identified using either the operator's hand or the obturator of an end-to-end anastomosis rectal tool. The bladder and the peritoneum are dissected off the anterior vaginal wall and any fascial tears are identified and repaired. the graft used for the procedure is synthetic polypropylene graft with the long arm 4–5 cm that will extend down the posterior vagina and a shorter end 2–3 cm that is secured to the anterior vaginal wall. Typically, rows of 2-0 polypropylene sutures are placed along the back wall and 2 rows are placed along the anterior. Once secured to the graft, the vault can be suspended to the sacral promontory with minimal tension. Prior to suspending to the apex, a culdoplasty should be performed to obliterate the cul-de-sac and prevent future enterocele formation. After the vault is suspended, the abdomen is copiously irrigated, and the peritoneum closed, the major complications related to the procedure are hemorrhage from sacral promontory and postoperative ileus the risk of bleeding can be minimized by using bone anchors on the sacral promontory.

Postoperative Details

Patients need to avoid any heavy lifting over 5 pounds for at least 6 weeks after surgery. At their 6-week postoperative visit the surgical site is assessed and if the area is well healed the patient is instructed to progressively return to their usual daily activities. Post-menopausal patients are instructed to use vaginal estrogen 1 g twice weekly to maintain integrity of the pelvic tissues. Patients are instructed to follow-up 3 months after they return to normal activities to assess the repair. Authors also continually follow to evaluate the integrity of the repair.

CONCLUSION

Pelvic reconstructive surgeons should be extremely familiar with evaluation and treatment of vaginal vault prolapse. Multiple techniques are available for the restoration of vaginal vault support, and most are very effective at suspending the vaginal apex. The primary challenge is identifying the vaginal vault in women with advanced degree of vaginal prolapse the surgical approach should be based on both patients' needs and surgeons' evaluation.

REFERENCES

1. Abrams P, Cardozo L, Fall M, et al. The standardisation of terminology of lower urinary tract function: report from the Standardisation Sub-committee of the International Continence Society. Neurourol Urodyn. 2002;21(2):167-78. doi: 10.1002/nau.10052.
2. McCall ML. Posterior culdoplasty: surgical correction of enterocele during vaginal hysterectomy: a preliminary report. Am J Obstet Gynaecol. 1957;10:595-602.

13 CHAPTER

Nadkarni's SEA Operation: Sleeve Surgery

Manohar Motwani, Kartikeya Bhagat

INTRODUCTION

- Dr Raman Mangesh Nadkarni, an astute Ob/Gyn specialist and an avid researcher, is a name lesser known in the field of Ob/Gyn.
- Somehow, the recognition he deserves in the annals of Ob/Gyn is lacking and out of proportion to the amount and kind of work he has done.
- This is a humble attempt at restoring the glory and the place in history that he richly deserves.
- Dr Nadkarni's Supravaginal Excision and Anastomosis (SEA) operation, the most rational surgery designed for young women with Supravaginal Elongation of the Cervix (SVEC) desirous of childbearing, is somehow lost in the labyrinths of the archives. It definitely deserves a re-look, a re-visit.

THE MAN AND HIS JOURNEY

- Dr Raman Mangesh Nadkarni was an alumnus of the Seth GS Medical College and KEM Hospital, Mumbai, Maharashtra. He was awarded MD, DGO (Obs/Gyne) in 1953. He worked at the ICMR and Nair Hospital, Mumbai as a Research Assistant for 2 years after graduation.
- He migrated to Ahmedabad and served the Sheth Vadilal Sarabhai Hospital, in the capacity of a Full Timer and later Honorary Professor for 30 years. His research continued in his Private Practice. He was an active Member and President of the Ahmedabad Ob/Gynec Society (AOGS) and served as the President of FOGSI in 1981 at Chandigarh.
- He devised and innovated multiple surgical procedures for problems related to the uterus, cervix, ovaries and the perineum. The most important and original surgery, he described was the SEA operation.

NADKARNI'S SUPRAVAGINAL EXCISION AND ANASTOMOSIS OF CERVIX OR THE SLEEVE SURGERY

Thought Processes and Experimental Work

- The most popular conservative surgery for the treatment of prolapse with an elongated cervix was the Fothergill's Manchester Operation at that time.

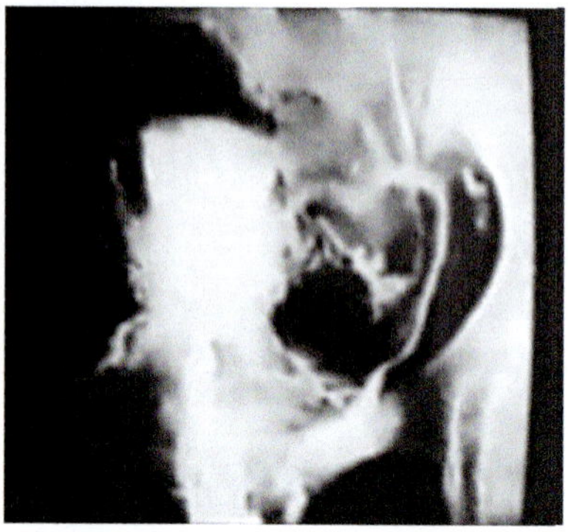

Fig. 1: Blood supply to the portio vaginalis with adequate collaterals.

- *His reservations*: Dr Nadkarni felt that the Fothergill's-Manchester operation was too radical for patients with pelvic organ prolapse (POP) with SVEC who were desirous of fertility because the 'cervical factor' necessary for fertility and normal sex life was sacrificed.
- He believed that the Fothergill's operation involved excision of the infravaginal portion of cervix when the problem was the SVEC in POP.
- *His aim:* Sleeve excision of the elongated middle part of the cervix and its reconstruction by anastomosing its proximal and distal ends so that cervical function would not be compromised significantly.
- *His experiments:* He studied the blood circulation of cervix extensively:
    - Angiographic study of the circulation in the parametrium revealed that the portio vaginalis has an independent blood supply with adequate collaterals **(Fig. 1)**.
    - Since bilateral ligation of uterine artery or anterior division of internal iliac artery and cervical encirclage did not result in sloughing of portio vaginalis in his experimental work, he concluded that excision of the supravaginal part of cervix should not disturb the circulation of portio vaginalis and will not cause sloughing.
    - His experiments with excision of the supravaginal portion of the cervix during vaginal hysterectomies established that the elongated endovaginal/endopelvic fascia has a loose attachment to the cervical tissue making dissection quite easy and bloodless. He observed that there was no color change in the portio vaginalis after experimental sleeve excision and anastomosis indicating undisturbed circulation.
    - *His conclusion:*
        - The elongation of the cervix was noticed below the level of the histological internal os and never affected the length of the isthmus.
        - The paracervical tissue below the histological internal os was loosely attached to the cervix (proved by injecting normal saline, which undergoes elongation).

- The portio vaginalis has significant blood supply and also has collaterals from lateral side.
- Excision of the supravaginal portion of the cervix and anastomosis is a safe and rewarding operation for cases of PoP with supravaginal elongation of cervix in childbearing age.

- He presented this work at:
  - "A preliminary report of 12 cases" Ob/Gyn Conference in Mumbai, 1979.
  - All India Ob/Gyn Congress at Bengaluru, 1980.
  - Video presentation in the XI World Ob/Gyn Congress at Berlin, 1985.

- *Principles/Steps of Surgery* **(Figs. 2 to 8)**:
  1. Dilatation of cervix upto No. 11 dilator.
  2. I-shaped incision on anterior vaginal wall.
  3. Bladder reflected up by a transverse incision at cervicovaginal junction
  4. Adrenaline saline injected in the pericervical fascia along sides of the cervix to be excised.
  5. Vertical incision on the pericervical fascia from the level of the anatomical internal os to just above the external os.
  6. Fascia undermined and separated from cervix so as to expose the column of the cervix and sleeve.
  7. Cervical column exposed and separated by blunt and rarely sharp dissection.
  8. Cervical column, i.e., the sleeve marked out—lower end above the attachment of the pubocervical ligament and the upper end quite below the histological internal os identified by firm attachment of fascia and the tendency to bleed while separating it. The sleeve to be cut at least 0.5 cm less than its actual elongation.

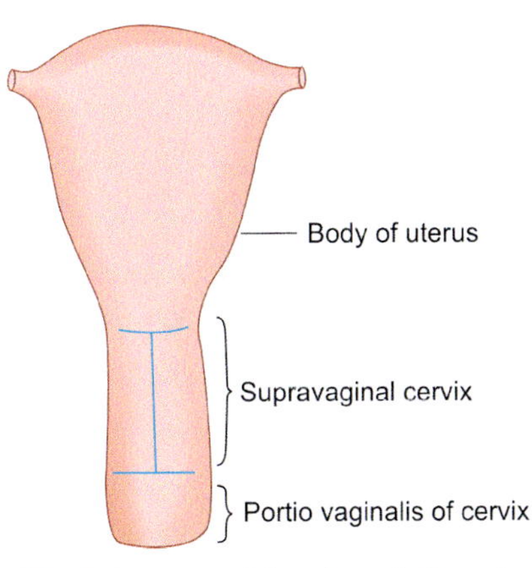

Fig. 2: Anatomy of the elongated cervix.

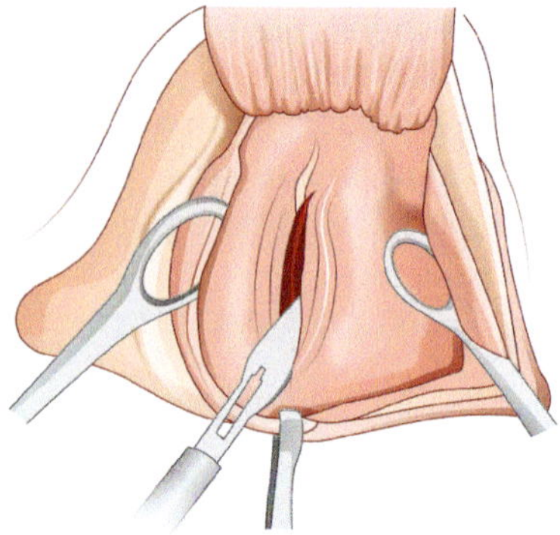

Fig. 3: Vertical incision on pericervical fascia.

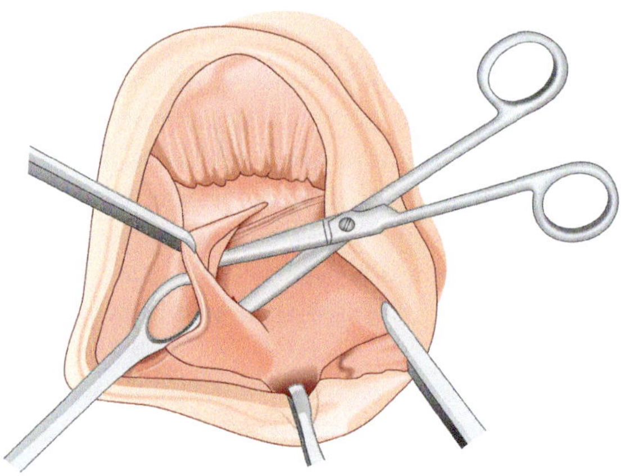

Fig. 4: Undermining and separation of pericervical fascia.

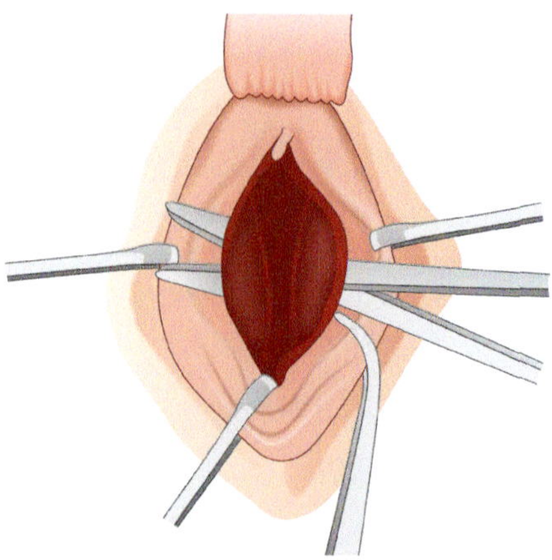

Fig. 5: Dissection and separation of the cervical sleeve.

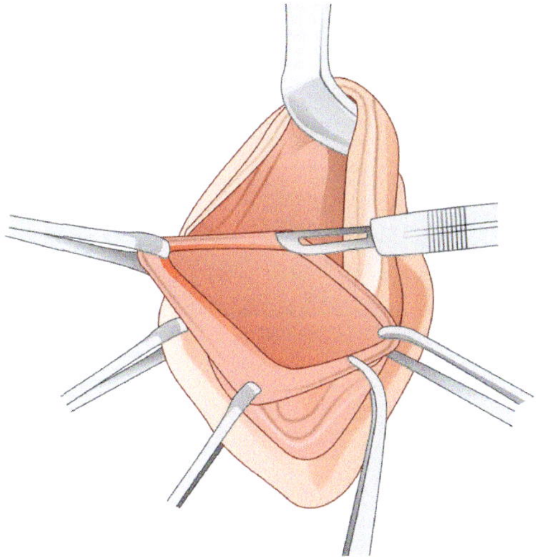

Fig. 6: Excision of elongated cervical sleeve.

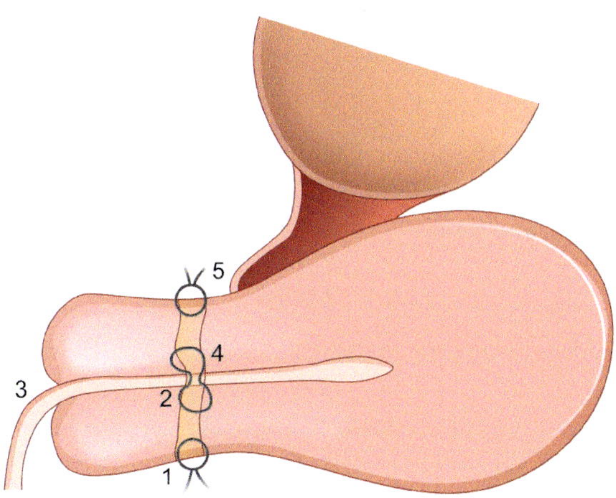

Fig. 7: Anastomosis of the proximal and distal portion in layers.

9. Anastomosis of the proximal and distal portion done in layers—endocervical mucosa sutured with 2-0 chromic catgut, cervical and pericervical outer fibrous layer sutured with Prolene no 1, interrupted sutures. Anastomosis covered by suturing the endopelvic fascia with Prolene 2-0.
10. Self-retaining Foley's catheter no. 14 (balloon inflated to 2 cc) kept as a stent in the cervical canal for 7 days.
11. Cervix and vagina assume a normal look after 3 weeks of surgery.

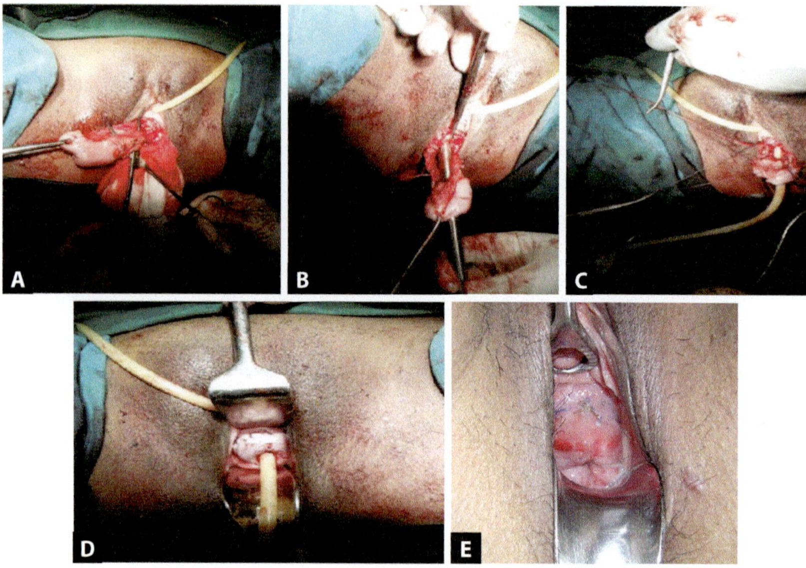

Figs. 8A to E: Postoperative day 14.
Courtesy: Drs Geeta Niyogi and Rahul Mayekar.

RESULTS

Till 1980, Dr Nadkarni performed 45 operations. There were 9 pregnancies: 4 had CS, 4 delivered vaginally, 1 had a mid-trimester abortion and 1 had a hysterectomy at a later date.

HOW THE WORLD LOOKS AT IT

- Dr RM Nadkarni never received the recognition he deserves for this surgery.
- The SEA operation was presented at the Ob/Gyn Conference in Bombay (1979) and the All India Ob/Gyn Conference at Bengaluru (1980) and Video Presentation at the World Congress of Ob/Gyn at Berlin (1985).

ANZJOG

Reproductive Performance Following Sleeve Excision Anastomosis Operation for Genital Prolapse

Gautam N. Allahbadia MD, FCPS, DGO, DFP, DNB

SUMMARY

Genital prolapse is a disorder of pelvic support and is one of the most frequent disorders encountered in our gynecological practice. Our social and cultural background predispose to this condition to occur at an age which is reported to be earlier than any part of the world. Over a period of 4 years,

1986–1989, 17 cases were studies in whom the sleeve excision anastomosis operation was carried out, either at the Lokmanya Tilak Municipal General Hospital, Sion, Mumbai, Maharashtra, India or in some other hospital. All these patients were either admitted in active labor or as cases of abortions or were being treated for infertility. The incidence of the cesarean section was 8.3%. There was 1 case of posterior wall rupture following previous sleeve excision anastomosis operation. The recurrence rate of prolapse in our series was only 7.7%. The sleeve excision anastomosis operation has given excellent anatomical and obstetric results in our study and future multicentric trials will be necessary to study its effect on subsequent fertility to arrive at any final conclusion.

CONCLUSION

- Dr Nadkarni's SEA operation is a very logical, rational and relatively simple surgery.
- It definitely merits a place in the surgical logarithm for treatment of POP.
- Its niche role is in well-selected case of SVEC in young patients desirous of childbearing, especially in the modern era, where laparoscopy seems to be the answer to most cases of genital prolapse in young patients.

ACKNOWLEDGMENT

- Dr RM Nadkarni's contribution to Gynecology and Obstetrics, complied by Dr Ramila Jain, published by Dr RM Nadkarni Medical Education and Research Trust
- Grateful and thankful to:
    - Dr Yashuben Patel (Ahmedabad), Dr Sarita Hattangadi (Mumbai)
    - Dr Geeta Niyogi (LTMGH, Mumbai), Dr Vivek Patkar (LTMGH, Mumbai), Dr Mohan Gadam (LTMGH, Mumbai), Dr Rahul Mayekar (LTMGH, Mumbai), Dr RM Saraogi (Mumbai)

14 CHAPTER

Native Tissue for Vaginal Apex Repair

Anil Sakhare

Pelvic organ prolapse (POP) is a broad term used to describe the prolapse of any of the three vaginal compartments: the anterior (cystocele), posterior (rectocele), and apical (uterine and vault prolapse). Up to 50% of women who have given birth may experience POP, and roughly one in nine women will require at least one surgery for it during their lifetime. Native tissue repair remains a fundamental approach in treating prolapse, especially given the ongoing debate about the safety and efficacy of using mesh. Over time, improvements in surgical techniques have been guided by a deep understanding of anatomy and surgical principles, alongside new insights gained from clinical research.

Pelvic organ prolapse occurs when the pelvic organs lose their support and start to bulge into the vagina.[1] The types of POP are named after the organ involved: a cystocele (anterior compartment prolapse) is when the bladder protrudes into the vagina; a rectocele (posterior compartment prolapse) involves the rectum pushing into the back of the vagina; and a vault prolapse (apical prolapse) happens when the top of the vagina falls into the lower part. Vault prolapse is frequently linked with an enterocele, which is the herniation of the small intestine into the vagina. "Vault prolapse" implies that the uterus is not present, whereas "uterine prolapse" indicates the uterus is still there.

POP impacts about 50% of women, leading to significant emotional distress and a decreased quality of life, while also placing a heavy financial burden on the healthcare system. The cost of treating POP in the US from 2005 to 2006 was over $300 million,[2] a figure expected to rise as the elderly female population grows. Current estimates suggest that POP affects between 3 and 6% of women.[3]

Parity is a significant risk factor for developing POP, with the risk increasing with each additional birth. Research by Mant et al. found that women who have had one childbirth are four times more likely to need hospitalization for POP compared to those who have not given birth, with this risk rising with each subsequent vaginal delivery.[4] Vaginal delivery is associated with a higher risk of POP compared to cesarean section. Larsson and his team discovered that 92.9% of women with POP had vaginal deliveries, while only 1.9% had cesarean sections. Lukacz et al. also noted that women who went into labor before having a cesarean section had a higher rate of POP compared to those who had an elective cesarean section without labor.[5]

Other risk factors for POP include aging, previous pelvic surgeries, chronic constipation, and obesity.[6,7]

Most POP surgeries use the patient's own tissue, but recurrence rates after native tissue repair can reach up to 29%. Some experts believe this failure rate is overstated, with actual rates between 9–15%.[8] As a result, surgeons have started using biological grafts and synthetic mesh to improve outcomes. While synthetic mesh can enhance anatomical results, it has also led to complications, prompting the FDA to issue safety warnings.[9,10] Given the current and projected prevalence of POP, along with the ongoing debate about mesh use, it is crucial for clinicians to be well informed about native tissue repair options for treating this condition.

Data from the OPTIMAL trial indicate that uterosacral ligament suspension and sacrospinous ligament fixation are equally effective for treating apical prolapse. However, some surgeons prefer McCall culdoplasty, which involves plicating the uterosacral ligaments. This technique provides direct visualization, either internally or externally, allowing for precise placement of apical support stitches and tightening the ligaments in the center of the vaginal cuff to help prevent enterocele formation. DeLancey's research highlights the various levels of support in the female pelvis and emphasizes the importance of apical support. It is essential to remember that anterior and posterior compartment prolapses often occur alongside apical prolapse, making treatment of the apex crucial for overall success.

EXTERNAL VS. INTERNAL McCALL SUTURES TECHNIQUE

Picture the open vaginal cuff following a vaginal hysterectomy or when addressing a vaginal vault prolapse post-hysterectomy. You can use either external or internal McCall sutures to support the vaginal apex.

With external sutures, you thread the suture through the vaginal cuff epithelium into the peritoneal cavity, incorporating the uterosacral ligaments and intervening peritoneum, and then bring it back out through the posterior cuff to tie it. Internal sutures involve placing the suture directly in the intraperitoneal space, securing the uterosacral ligaments and peritoneum, and tying it off internally. Sometimes, a combination of both techniques is employed.

For external sutures, I use 0-polyglactin. This choice is intentional, as these sutures dissolve over time and would not remain in the vaginal cavity. I generally place at least two external sutures, starting with the deepest one at the vaginal cuff, which should be the most distal uterosacral stitch.

Subsequent sutures are placed progressively closer to the vaginal cuff and the ends of the ligamentous stumps, beginning with the deepest stitch, and working towards the cuff.

I also place one or two internal sutures, which can be either delayed, absorbable, or permanent. These are placed between the external sutures, tied off internally in the intraperitoneal space. Permanent sutures may be used here due to their location and the fact they will be tied off internally (*see* **Figs. 1 and 2**).

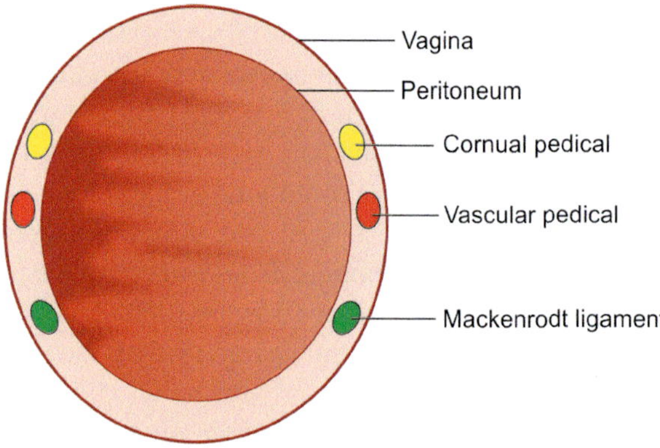

Fig. 1: The open vaginal cuff following a vaginal hysterectomy or when addressing a vaginal vault prolapse post-hysterectomy.

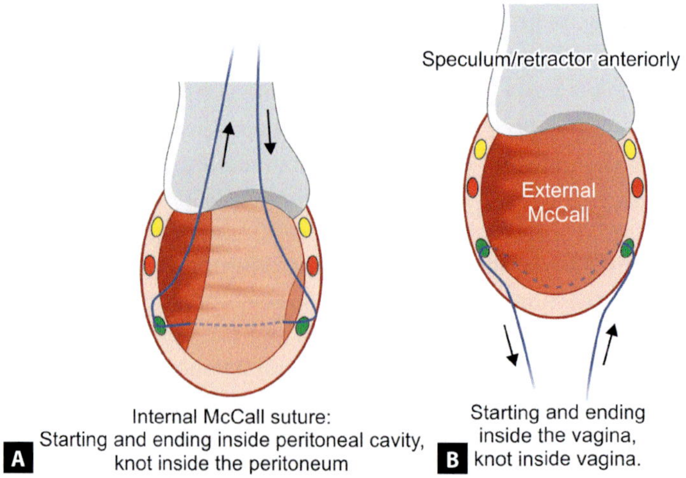

Figs. 2A and B: Internal McCall suture. (A) Starting and ending inside peritoneal cavity, knot inside the peritoneum; (B) Starting and ending inside the vagina, knot inside vagina.

UTEROSACRAL LIGAMENT SUSPENSION TECHNIQUE

When performing uterosacral ligament stitches, there is a known risk of kinking or injuring the ureter. Thus, cystoscopy is essential to ensure safety during the procedure. Securing apical support allows you to build effective anterior and posterior repairs on this foundation. It is crucial to clearly define the space between the ureter and rectum on each side when performing uterosacral ligament suspension. Elevating the cardinal pedicle and medially retracting the rectum can help with this. Remember, the ligament descends toward the sacrum when the patient is supine, so it is important to follow this trajectory to avoid injury. Additionally, be cautious not to plicate too deeply, as this could lead to defecatory dysfunction.

Uterosacral ligament suspension (USLS) is one of the most commonly performed native tissue procedures for vault prolapse. Traditionally, this involves entering the peritoneal cavity to locate the uterosacral ligaments. However, an extraperitoneal approach has also been described.[11] In this technique, sutures are placed bilaterally through the uterosacral ligaments at the level of the ischial spine, including the lateral pubocervical and rectovaginal fascia. Tying these sutures helps elevate and anchor the vaginal cuff to the uterosacral ligaments,[12] and it also addresses any associated enterocele defects.

There is a significant risk of ureteral injury with vaginal USLS. Contemporary studies comparing laparoscopic and vaginal approaches to USLS suggest that both methods have similar clinical outcomes and complication rates, though laparoscopic procedures have a lower rate of ureteral injury. Regardless of the approach used, intraoperative cystoscopy is crucial for detecting any potential ureteral issues.

For a successful repair, ensure that your procedure restores continuity between the anterior endopelvic fascia and the fascia and ligaments at the vaginal apex. This step is key to effectively addressing anterior compartment prolapse.

SACROSPINOUS LIGAMENT SUSPENSION

Sacrospinous ligament suspension (SSLS) is a widely used transvaginal method for treating apical prolapse. This approach gained prominence with the advent of transvaginal mesh kits. Both anterior and posterior techniques for accessing the sacrospinous ligament have been developed. During the procedure, sutures are placed carefully through the sacrospinous ligament, ensuring they are positioned medially to the ischial spine to avoid the pudendal neurovascular bundle. Utilizing a suture device, like the First Pass Mini instrument—often used by orthopedic surgeons in arthroscopies—can simplify this process. I have found this tool particularly effective for passing the suture.

Once the sutures are in place, the vaginal muscularis is secured to the sacrospinous ligament. It is worth considering unilateral suspension on the right side, as the sigmoid colon and rectum on the left may present challenges. Common complications include hemorrhage and gluteal pain, which typically resolve on their own, as well as potential bladder or rectal injuries.

Given the recent FDA ban on transvaginal mesh for POP and the public's often negative perception of mesh—sometimes influenced by misleading media reports—it is crucial for gynecologic surgeons to focus on mastering or revisiting native tissue repair techniques. While not without their limitations, these techniques provide a viable non-mesh option for many patients.

REFERENCES

1. Wein AJ, Kavoussi LR, Campbell MF, Walsh PC. Campbell-Walsh urology. 10th edn, 2012. Elsevier Saunders, Philadelphia, PA.
2. Sung VW, Washington B, Raker CA. Costs of ambulatory care related to female pelvic floor disorders in the United States. Am J Obstet Gynecol. 2010;202(5):483 e1-4. doi:10.1016/j. ajog.2010.01.015.
3. Barber MD, Maher C. Epidemiology and outcome assessment of pelvic organ prolapse. Int Urogynecol J. 2013;24(11):1783-90. Doi: 10.1007/s00192-013-2169-9.
4. Mant J, Painter R, Vessey M. Epidemiology of genital prolapse: observations from the Oxford family planning association study. Br J Obstet Gynaecol. 1997;104(5):579-85.
5. Lukacz ES, Lawrence JM, Contreras R, Nager CW, Luber KM. Parity, mode of delivery, and pelvic floor disorders. Obstet Gynecol. 2006;107(6):1253-60. doi:10.1097/01.AOG.0000218096.54169.34.
6. Swift S, Woodman P, O'Boyle A, Kahn M, Valley M, Bland D, et al. Pelvic organ support study (POSST): the distribution, clinical definition, and epidemiologic condition of pelvic organ support defects. Am J Obstet Gynecol. 2005;192(3):795-806. Doi: 10.1016/j. ajog.2004.10.602.
7. Kudish BI, Iglesia CB, Sokol RJ, Cochrane B, Richter HE, Larson J, et al. Effect of weight change on natural history of pelvic organ prolapse. Obstet Gynecol. 2009;113(1):81-8. doi:10.1097/AOG.0b013e318190a0dd
8. Karram MM. OBG Management. 2020;32:2.
9. Nguyen JN, Burchette RJ. Outcome after anterior vaginal prolapse repair: a randomized controlled trial. Obstet Gynecol. 2008;111(4): 891-8. doi:10.1097/AOG.0b013e31816a2489.
10. FDA Safety Communication. UPDATE on serious complications associated with transvaginal placement of surgical mesh for pelvic organ prolapse, 2011.
11. Ow LL, Walsh CE, Rajamaheswari N, Dwyer PL. Technique of extraperitoneal uterosacral ligament suspension for apical suspension. Int Urogynecol J. 2016;27(4):637-9. doi:10.1007/s00192-015-2873-8.
12. Karram M, Goldwasser S, Kleeman S, Steele A, Vassallo B, Walsh P. High uterosacral vaginal vault suspension with fascial reconstruction for vaginal repair of enterocele and vaginal vault prolapse. Am J Obstet Gynecol. 2001;185(6):1339-42. discussion 42-3 doi:10.1067/mob.2001.119077.

15 CHAPTER

Manchester-Fothergill Procedure

Mohan A Gadam

INTRODUCTION

Manchester-Fothergill repair is essentially a conservative surgery for prolapsed uterus in a young patient who is keen on preserving her menstrual and childbearing functions. It is used commonly done in Europe for this purpose, and also invented in Europe.

HISTORY

- The first conservative operation to be described for the treatment of genital prolapse was that devised by Archibald Donald and William Fothergill: the Manchester operation.
- The Manchester operation was later modified by VN Shirodkar who described uterosacral advancement operation; in this modification, cervix is not amputated.

INDICATIONS FOR THE PROCEDURE

Young patient who is keen on preserving her menstrual and childbearing functions and she has following conditions fulfilled:

- She has a uterovaginal prolapse, preferably not more than 2nd or 3rd degree.
- Uterocervical length >3 inches and not more than 5 inches.
- May or may not have cystocele and/or rectocele.
- Any other pelvic pathology ruled out which contraindicate surgery.

PREOPERATIVE WORKUP

- A thorough general, systemic and pelvic examination is done to satisfy all the indications and to rule out contraindications for the procedure.
- Patients should be thoroughly investigated for fitness for surgery and anesthesia.

SURGICAL DETAILS

- Under suitable anesthesia, the patient is brought to the edge of the table.
- She is given a dorsal lithotomy position.
- Parts are painted and draped.
- Labial stitches are taken to keep labia out of the operative field.
- Cervix is held with two vulsellum or Allis forceps.
- The degree of descent is judged along with the presence of cystocele and/or rectocele.
- One proceeds with precise steps of Manchester-Fothergill's repair.

The essential steps of Fothergill's repair are:

- Preliminary dilatation and curettage
- Ligation of descending cervical vessels on either side so as to avoid intraoperative hemorrhage
- Amputation of cervix
- Advancement of Mackenrodt ligament in front of cervix
- Covering the raw area of the cervical stump with anterior and the posterior Sturmdorf stitches.
- Anterior colporrhaphy
- Posterior colpoperineorrhaphy

Dilatation and Curettage

The uterocervical length is measured, and the cervix is dilated with rapid, serial metallic dilators to around 10–12 numbers.

Dilatation serves two purposes:

1. It facilitates curettage.
2. It helps in taking proper Sturmdorf sutures.

Curettage is an essential step as we can send the tissue for histopathology and we also try to ensure that this patient will not bleed in the next 12–15 days of postoperative period. It is at this time that patients can have secondary hemorrhage, and hence there should be no confusion between the two conditions.

- After D&C is done, saline adrenaline (1 in 100,000 dilution) is infiltrated in the area where one is likely to take the incision.
- Anterior incision is taken around 1/2 to 1 inch above external os (This is in fact a step which is deviation from standard Manchester-Fothergill repair where in the anterior and the posterior incisions were taken depending on four Fothergill's points).
- If there is an elongated Portio Vaginalis of cervix, then the anterior incision needs to be taken higher up in the vicinity of bladder sulcus.
- This becomes a necessary step to avoid excessive bleeding and to easily reach the peritoneum of anterior cul-de-sac.

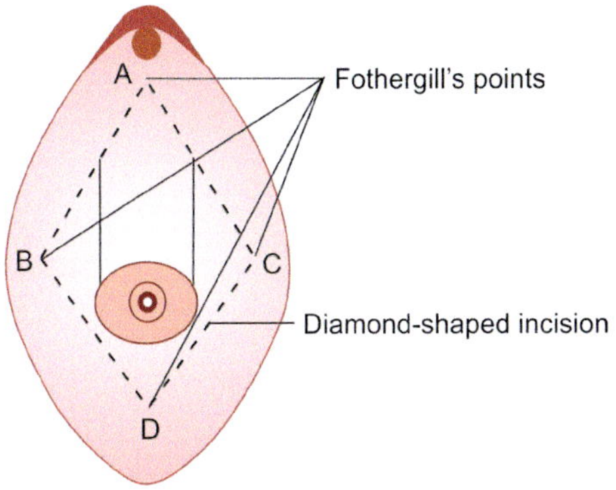

Fig. 1: Exposure of anterior and posterior surfaces of the cervix.

Bladder Dissection/Exposing the Anterior and Posterior Lip of Cervix/Preparing for Cervical Amputation

- With traction and sharp or blunt dissection (I am a strong proponent of sharp rather than blunt dissection).
- If the plane is correct, it will be a treat to watch and it is the ease at which we can reach the anterior uterovesical fold of peritoneum is wonderful.
- If one's plane sense is correct, then in my opinion sharp dissection should be the gold standard.
- However, I am not an authority on this subject and hence we recommend to go by surgeon's preferences.
  In Fothergill's repair, there is no need to open anterior cul-de-sac and in fact even the posterior cul-de-sac. It is extremely important to avoid soiling of peritoneal cavity thereby minimizing the potential risk of postoperative infection and peritonitis.
- Exposure of anterior and posterior surfaces of the cervix becomes essential as it will facilitate amputation of cervix and advancing the Mackenrodt ligament anteriorly **(Fig. 1)**.

FOTHERGILL'S POINTS

The original Manchester repair described four Fothergill's points. As shown in **Figure 1**, point A is below external urethral meatus in the midline depending on the grade of cystocele. Point B and C are in the lateral fornices around 1.5 inches away from external os, and Point D is in the posterior fornix in the region of posterior cul-de-sac. After having marked these points, the vaginal flaps are excised between these points to complete the above step.

CARDINAL LIGAMENTS

- Mackenrodt or the cardinal ligaments are then identified on either side.
- Each one is clamped, cut and transfixed doubly and the ligature is kept long and equal.

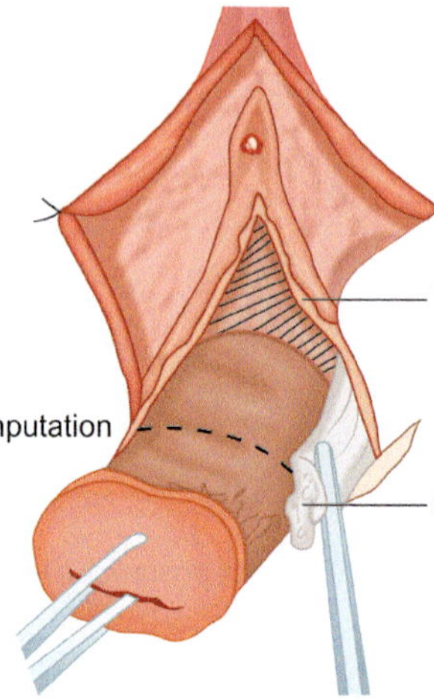

Fig. 2: Cystole repair.

Descending Cervical

- It is important that descending cervical vessels on both sides should be ligated before attempting cervical amputation.
- Descending cervical artery is the major vessel supplying the entire cervix and once it is ligated on either side, cervix becomes reasonably avascular and hence post-amputation intraoperative blood loss is certainly minimized.
- A delayed absorbable suture material (Polyglycolic or polygalactic acid: Dexon or Vicryl) is number 1 on 40 mm sought cutting or trocar point, eyeless needle is used to take descending cervical.
- Care should be taken to avoid injury directly to the vessel, and hence the medial transfixation suture should be placed well within the substance of the cervix **(Fig. 2)**.
- The urinary bladder along with portion of pubo-vasico-cervical fascia is then pushed up by sharp and blunt dissection and the anterior surface of the cervix is exposed completely.
- Bladder base is then buttressed with a series of delayed absorbable sutures and the cystocele is taken care.

CERVICAL AMPUTATION

Amputation of cervix is the next step which is crucial for optimum results of this surgery **(Fig. 3)**.

The following steps are usually adhered to while performing amputation of cervix:

- Amputation is required only when the cervix is elongated and thus needs to be shortened.

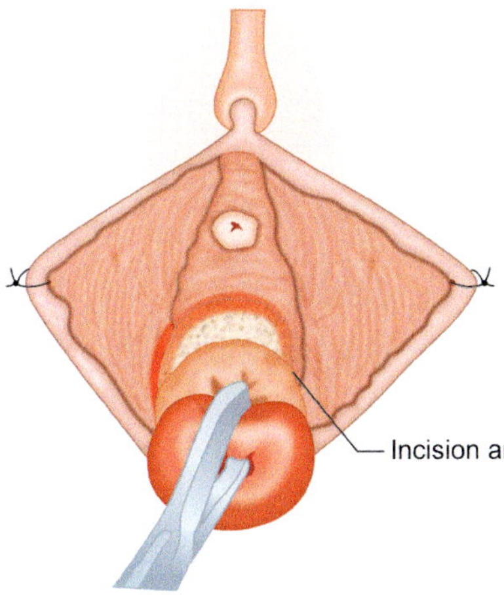

Fig. 3: Cervical amputation

- A 12-number blade on BP handle is used for this procedure.
- Alternatively, a monopolar cutting current can also be used to achieve similar results (We avoid using monopolar current as the tissue necrosis giving rise to irritating postoperative discharge is often bothersome).
- A desired level of amputation is predefined. One needs to keep at least 2.00–2.50 cm of cervix so as to preserve adequate number of endo-cervical glands for fertility preservation.
- If one is very harsh on removing bigger length of cervix, in that case we may be inviting iatrogenic subfertility and cervical insufficiency in future pregnancies.
- The level to which the amputation is required to be carried out is marked on the cervix anteriorly and posteriorly.
- One start amputating the cervix, as we go down, keep the blade inclined thereby beveling the cervix while going down (This is a deviation from original Fothergill repair so as to ensure better shape to the cervix which will mimic normal shape).
- A Guillotine amputation in fact may not give original shape, hence the change.
- After the amputation is over, it will be necessary to ensure that the raw area is not bleeding, and all the bleeding points are cauterized thoroughly.
- Often this is the cause of secondary hemorrhage which usually manifest within 12–15 days postoperative phase.

  Advancement of Cardinal (Mackenrodt Ligament) Ligaments
  - Mackenrodt ligaments on either side are bought in front of the cervix, crossed and transfixed to anterior wall of cervix.
  - Final tying of the knots is not done at this time, as certain precautions are to be observed while tying, as the uterus and the cervix need to

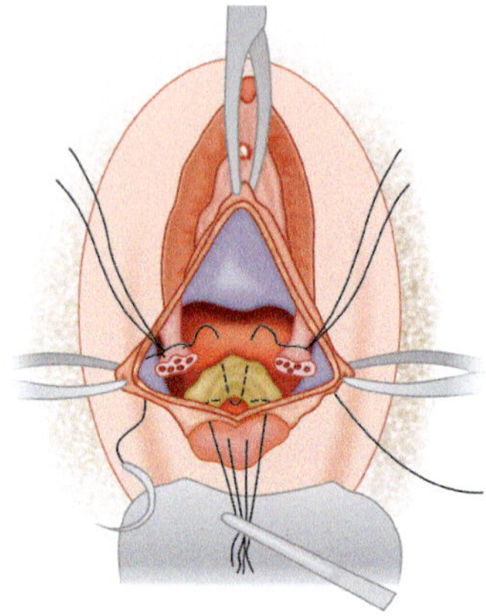

Fig. 4: Sturmdorf sutures or Fothergill stitch.

be raised up in the pelvis and then the sutures are tied. This is done to ensure that the uterus and the cervix remain pulled up after the surgery.

- Hence this procedure is often done after taking the posterior Sturmdorf suture.

Sturmdorf Sutures or Fothergill Stitch (Fig. 4)

Posterior Sturmdorf is taken first:

- Delayed absorbable number 1 suture is selected on 40 mm eyeless needle.
- The needle is passed through the central portion of the edge on posterior flap and the ligature is kept long and equal.
- The needle on one edge is then passed through dilated cervix and brought out on the posterior flap, around 1–1.5 cm away from the edge and 1 cm away from midline.
- This procedure is repeated at the second end of the suture.
- Both the sutures are then tied to each other, taking care that the uterus remains elevated while tying **(Figs. 5A to C)**.

Fothergill's Key Suture

- This suture is for anterior lips.
- The suture enters the vaginal skin at the level of Fothergill's lateral point and transfixes the cut cardinal ligament pedicles.
- The needle then passes from without inwards through the full thickness of the anterior cervical tissue near midline at 12 o'clock.
- The needle is now repassed from within outwards and through cardinal ligament pedicle of the opposite side and finally out at the opposite lateral Fothergill's point.

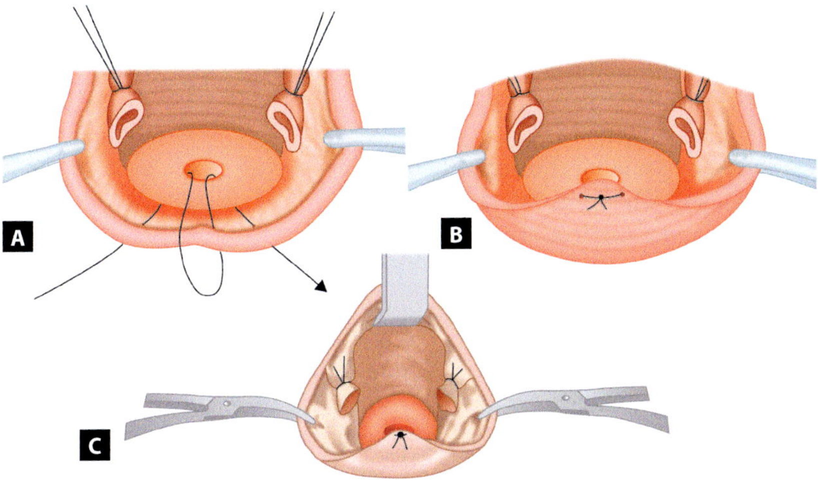

Figs. 5A to C: (A) Vaginal flap with cut ends of Mackenrodt ligament seen with amputated cervix and posterior Sturmdorf being taken; (B) Posterior Sturmdorf stitch covering entire posterior raw area on the cervix; (C) Posterior Sturmdorf.

- These two are then tied together in anterior midline.
- The net result is that the cardinal ligaments are approximated in the midline on anterior cervix and the raw area of the amputated cervix is covered with vaginal flap, thereby avoiding anterior Surmdorf.

Anterior Sturmdorf Sutures

- Anterior Sturmdorf is taken only if Fothergill suture is not taken.
- Procedure of anterior Sturmdorf is similar to that of posterior Sturmdorf and hence need not be repeated.

Lateral Sturmdorf Sutures

- Lateral Sturmdorf is not described in original Fothergill surgery. However, many surgeons or gynecologists strongly believe in it. I am also a staunch proponent of lateral Sturmdorf suture.
- As our experience for last 40 years on lateral Sturmdorf is good and thus we also advocate it to all our students.
- We prefer to do it whenever we find that the raw area on the lateral aspect cervix is not covered with a vaginal flap.
- The shape of the neocervix after the surgery is excellent, it appears like an appropriate anatomical reconstruction is done.

To conclude Manchester-Fothergill repair is an excellent conservative operation for uterine prolapse, in a young patient who is keen on preserving menstrual and childbearing functions.

The learning curve in slightly longer and many are not well trained in this procedure. Hence, the frequency with which this procedure is done is gradually going down. Besides, many alternatives are available for this procedure like:

- Modified Fothergill's repair
- Shirodkar's modification of Fothergill's repair
- Shirodkar's abdominal sling surgery
- BN Purandar cervicopexy
- Virkud sling
- Khanna sling
- Soonawala's sling
- Laparoscopic sling surgery

It is, however, mandatory for all of us to learn the technique and to keep ourselves well educated in this dying art, as this a wonderful procedure.

SUGGESTED READING

1. Manchester-Fothergill Procedure and Vaginal Wall Prolapse Repair. Von Voigtlander Womens Hospital, Mochigan
2. NIH ncbi.nim.nih.gov.
3. Te Linde's Operative Gynecology.
4. Wikipedia.org > WIKI > Manchester operation

16 CHAPTER

Debulking Techniques in Vaginal Hysterectomy

Mukesh Rathi

INTRODUCTION

Historically, debulking or volume reduction techniques have been described way back in the late 19th and mid-20th century by various gynecological surgeons, like Amussat, Czerney, Muller, Pryor, Lash and many others. The aim basically was to remove the uterus by the least invasive, vaginal route.[1]

INDICATIONS FOR DEBULKING

Whenever the size or the mobility of the uterus are a hinderance for sheering of the parametrial attachments, or delivery of the fibroid or uterus, by way of limitation of space or descent, then one needs to adopt the debulking techniques.

PRINCIPLES OF DEBULKING

Principle is gradual volume reduction so that the big size uterus/fibroids, adnexal mass can be delivered out or induce the giveaway of the uterine muscular wall, to facilitate gentle delivery.[2]

CRITERIA FOR DECIDING THE APPROACH

- *Clinical examination:* Assessment of the laxity of vagina, size, mobility, descent of the uterus, the number and location of the fibroids.
- Added factors like the previous lower (uterine) segment cesarean section (LSCS) or any uterine surgeries
- *USG:* For volume of the uterus, mapping the fibroids, associated adnexal pathology.
- *Examination under anesthesia:* For mobility, size, and descent
- Surgeon's experience backed up by the patient's willingness.[3]

Contraindications

- Malignancy must be ruled out.
- When the transverse axis of the uterus is more than the longitudinal axis[4] **(Fig. 1)** (Banyan-tree appearance)

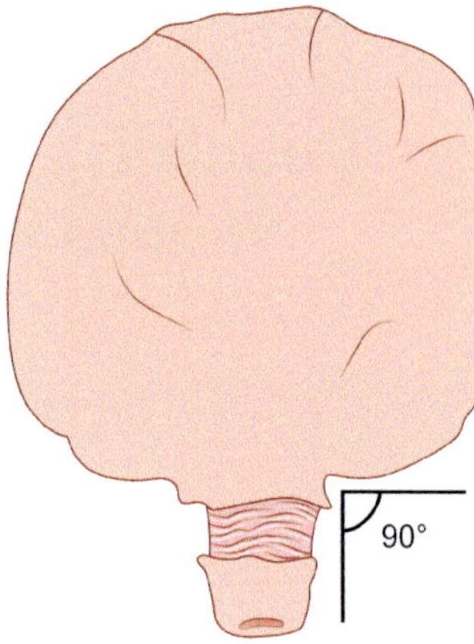

Fig. 1: The transverse axis of the uterus is more than the longitudinal axis.

Precautions

- Bladder should be empty/catheterized.
- Bladder and rectum secured under the respective anterior and posterior retractors.
- Avoid cluttering of the instruments or retractors.
- Morcellation should begin only after securing the uterine vascular bundle and under vision.
- Should know when to abandon.

VARIOUS TECHNIQUES OF DEBULKING[3]

Bisection/Hemisection

After the uterine vascular bundle is secured, steady traction is applied on the uterus and an incision is taken right from the cervix, vertically upwards, through the anterior and posterior wall. This induces give away of the myometrial muscle fibers and the uterus descend. Works well for upto 10–12 weeks size uterus[5,6] **(Fig. 2)**.

Transection

Here the uterus is cut transverse, so as to give more space to tackle the adnexal tissues or to reach the fibroid.

Pryor's Technique (Anterior Wedge Morcellation)

Uterus is bisected till as high as possible. After that, the wedges of the uterine tissue are cut anteriorly from the edges of the midline incision. The edges are further pulled down and similar wedges are cut from the part that descends, till the fundus is reached. Myomas on the way are enucleated. Works well when the POD is obliterated[7] **(Fig. 3)**.

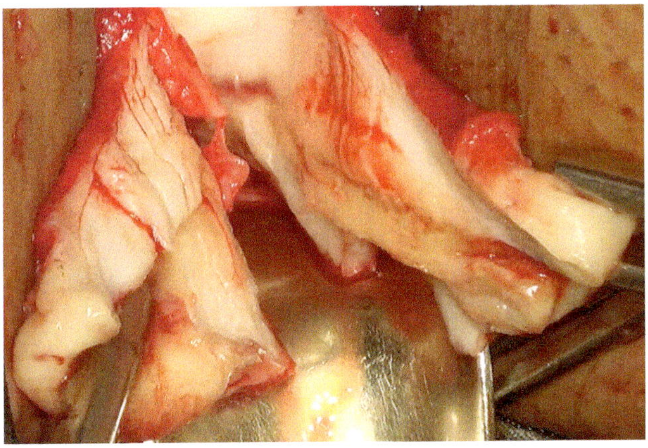

Fig. 2: Bisection.

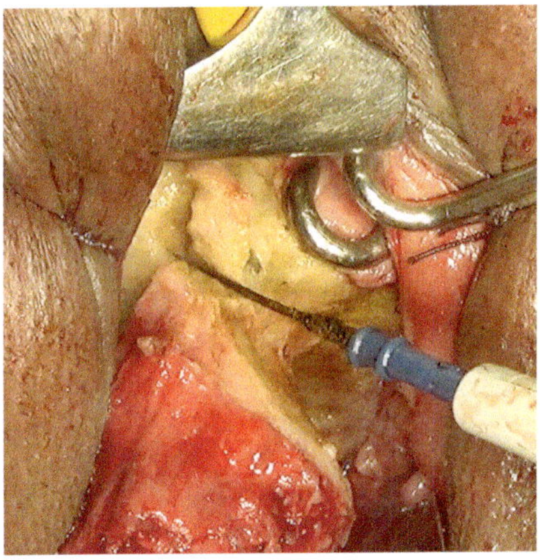

Fig. 3: Wedge morcellation.

Anteroposterior Wedge Resection

Cut the chunks of myometrium through the entire wall using the tenaculum or myoma screws, with the apex of the wedge digging into the substance of the uterine tissue, creating a sort of tunnel so that the walls collapse on each other, giving space for further progression.

Lash's Technique (Coring)

Well suited for elongated globular uteri or when subpubic angle is narrow. Circumferential incisions are taken serially on the myometrium, just below the serosa. This causes the inversion of serosa and myometrium above. Similar serial incisions are taken to deliver the uterus in a process like peeling a banana[8] **(Fig. 4)**.

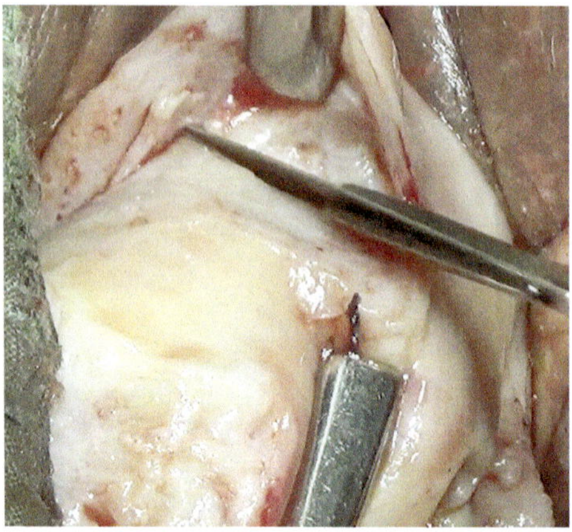

Fig. 4: Coring lash and lash.

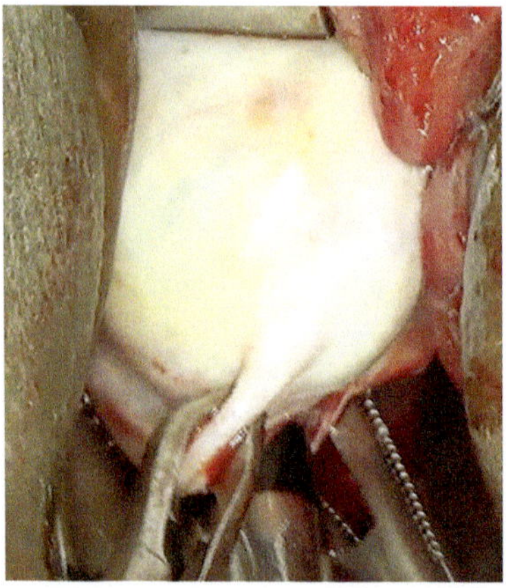

Fig. 5: Suction aspiration of big dermoid.

Debulking of the Benign Adnexal Cystic Masses

After the uterus is removed, traction is applied in the downward and outward direction on the cornual pedicle to bring the cyst in view and a small pack is pushed behind the cyst. Depending upon the size, a Veress needle or a 5-mm laparoscopic trochar-cannula is pushed in the cyst. Suction is applied through the needle or a suction cannula, that drains the entire cyst. The cyst drops into the field of surgery cystectomy or oopherectomy can be done as per the need[9,10] **(Fig. 5)**.

REFERENCES

1. Wasson MN, Butler KA, Temkit M, Magrina JF. Necessity of morcellation at time of vaginal hysterectomy. J Minim Invasive Gynecol. 2015;22(6S):S12. doi: 10.1016/j.jmig.2015.08.038.

2. Dubuisson J, Veit-Rubin N. Uterine volume and vaginal hysterectomy: interest and limits of uterine morcellation. Gynecol Obstet Fertil. 2016;44(3):175-80. doi: 10.1016/j.gyobfe.2016.01.008. Epub 2016 Mar 7.
3. Wasson M DO. Prognostic factors for morcellation during vaginal hysterectomy. Obstetrics & Gynecology. 2016;127(4):752-7. doi: 10.1097/AOG.0000000000001346.
4. Lash AF. A method of reducing the size of the uterus in vaginal hysterectomy. Am J Obstet and Gynaecol. 1941;42:452-8.
5. Sahen Y Vaginal hysterectomy and oopherectomy in women with 12–20 weeks size uterus. Acta Obstet Gynecol Scand. 2007;86:1359-69.
6. Quinlan D Vaginal hysterectomy in enlarged uterus: a report of 85 cases. J Obstet and Gynaecology Can. 2010;32:980-3
7. Nazah I, Robin F Comparison between bisection/morcellation and myometrial coring for reducing large uteri during vaginal hysterectomy or LAVH: results of a randomized prospective study. Acta Obstet Gynecol Scand. 2003;82:1037-42.
8. Sheth SS. Broad ligament myomectomy at vaginal hysterectomy without laparoscopic assistance. L Gynaecological Surgery. 2007;23 :133-42.
9. Sheth SS. Preoperative sonographic estimation of uterine volume: an aid to determine the route of hysterectomy. J Gynaecological Surgery. 2002:18:13-22.
10. Sheth SS. Adnexectomy for benign pathology at vaginal hysterectomy without laparoscopic assistance. Brit Journal of Obstet and Gynaecol. 2002;109:1401-5.

17

CHAPTER

Uterosacral Ligament as Native Tissue Support

Uma Rani Swain

INTRODUCTION

The uterosacral ligaments are essential components of the pelvic organ support system, playing a significant role in pelvic organ prolapse including vault prolapse. These strong supportive structures connect the cervix to the sacrum. Elongation and stretching of uterosacral ligaments are always considered as secondary to the ineffective pelvic floor to support the pelvic organs and also fails to sustain intra-abdominal pressure.[1]

Uterosacral ligament measures approximately 12–14 cm in length and arises from the lower lateral borders of the sacrum and coccyx, forming multiple tough fibers that merge to create robust, thick ligaments. This rod-like structure runs retroperitoneally, maintaining close proximity to the pelvic ureter in its course towards cervix. The ligaments form an inverted V-shaped with their counterparts at the insertion to posterior Cx. Due to their extended pelvic trajectory and firm attachment to the pelvic fascia, they stand as prominent cord-like structures in a curvilinear fashion just lateral to rectum. They delineate and separate the lateral groove of the rectum from the ureter on each side and can easily be picked up during pelvic procedures **(Fig. 1)**.

HISTOLOGICAL CONFIGURATION OF THE UTEROSACRAL LIGAMENTS (USL)

The uterosacral ligaments are thick, band-like structures composed of condensed connective tissue, smooth muscle, nerve fibers (including

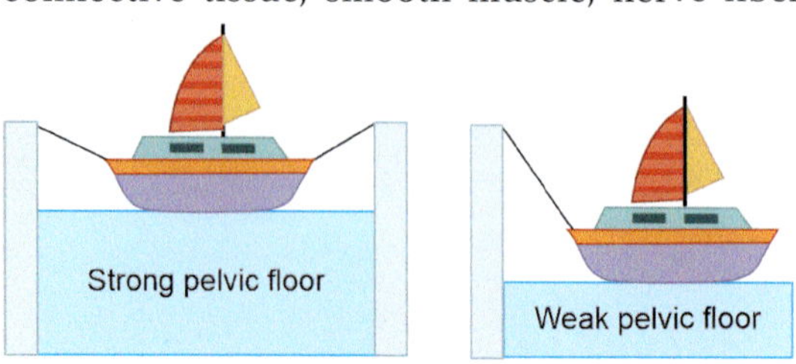

Fig. 1: Strong and weak pelvic floor.

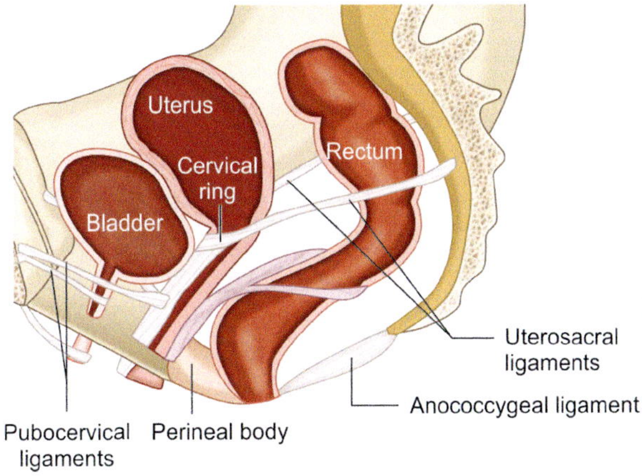

Fig. 2: Configuration of the uterosacral ligaments.

hypogastric and pelvic nerves), synaptic nodes, blood vessels, and fatty tissue. This composition provides the necessary strength to support the genital organs in their proper position **(Fig. 2)**.

The USL is divided into three segments:

1. *Distal:* 2–3 cm in length, attached to the cervix.
2. *Intermediate*: 5 cm long, running medial to the ischial spine.
3. *Proximal:* 5–6 cm long, in the form of ligamentous fibers attached to the lateral wall of the lower sacrum and coccyx.

The ischial spine is invariably positioned lateral to the intermediate segment of USL and guide as a light house, although the exact location of ligament fluctuates on few occasions. Both the cervical and intermediate segments of USL exhibited remarkable strength and can successfully hold 17 kg of weight before succumbing to failure. This highlights their substantial load-bearing capability **(Figs. 3 and 4)**.[2]

THE ROLE OF AUTOLOGOUS TISSUE SUPPORT

The uterosacral ligament (USL) plays a crucial role in maintaining uterine position and flexibility, more so during increase intra-abdominal pressure. As it also closely adhered to the apex of vagina before ending at Cx, it also supports the vault in post-hysterectomy case.

Apical suspension is considered to be the major step in prolapse repair. Suspension procedures are based on the principle of fixing the prolapse viscera to a tough structure-like ligament present inside the pelvis. The commonly selected native tissue is sacrospinous ligaments, and uterosacral ligaments if done vaginally, abdominally anterior longitudinal ligaments and pectineal ligaments. In the later procedure, synthetic mesh is used which acts like a new strong ligament to support the vault. In contrast, in vaginal

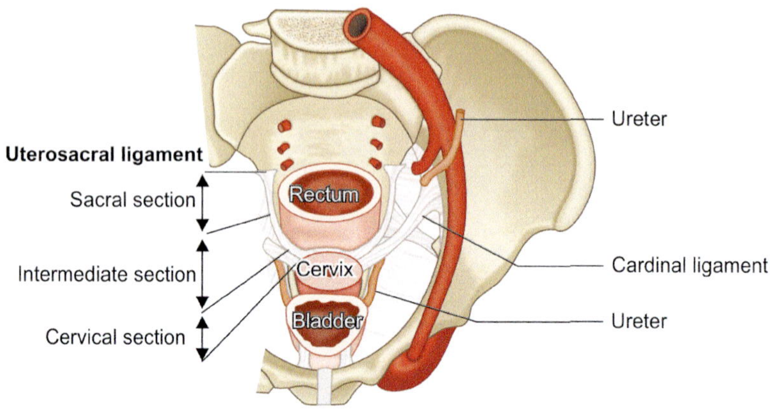

Fig. 3: A schematic diagram of the pelvis viewed from above showing the three parts of the uterosacral ligament and its relations with the cardinal ligament near the cervix.

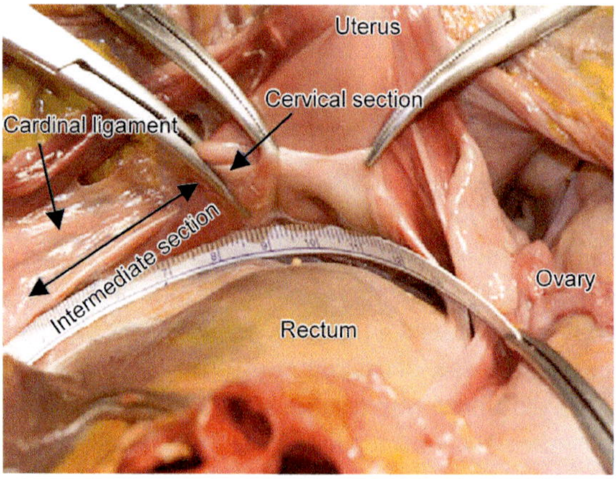

Fig. 4: Ligaments and supports of uterus and the parts of USL.

procedures because of native tissue, we get equally effective results and free of foreign body related complications like erosion, rejection and infection, etc. At the same time, it enjoys all advantages of natural passage surgery.[3]

Evidence of USL as Support

- In vault prolapse, a distinct dimple can be observed at the apex of the vault, which clearly signifies the USL's connection to the lateral angle of the vault.
- During the hysterectomy, with tension at angle of vault, the trajectory of the USL can be distinctly felt even visualized ascending beneath the pelvic peritoneum posteriorly.

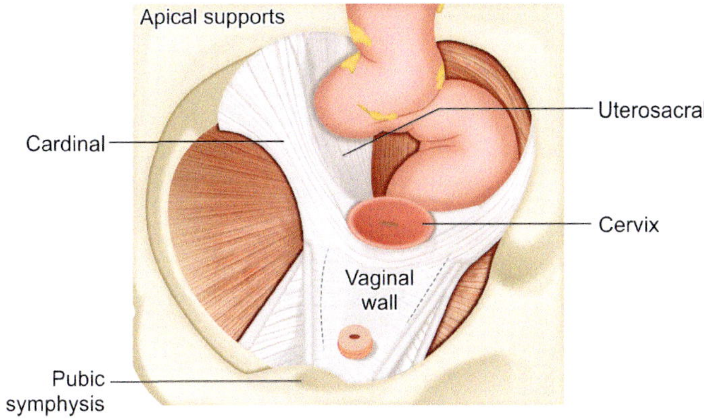

Fig. 5: High uterosacral ligament suspension (HUSLS).

- As pelvic organ prolapse (POP) progresses, the distal segment of the USL may stretch or partially denuded at places but the remaining upper segments remain unaffected in terms of length and strength.
- This understanding underpins the principles of the high uterosacral ligament suspension (HUSLS) procedure, which aims to restore pelvic organ support effectively **(Fig. 5)**.

RELATIONSHIP OF URETER TO USL

The ureter, a hollow tubular structure, runs parallel to the uterosacral ligament (USL) in the lower two-thirds of its pelvic course. While ascending the two structures begin to diverge from each other. At the distal end, the ureter is located approximately 1.5–2.5 cm from the USL, while in the upper segment, this distance increases to about 4–5 cm. This anatomical relationship suggests that the risk of ureteric injury during surgical procedures is significantly greater in McCall's culdoplasty procedure than in high uterosacral ligament suspension (HUSLS), due to its close proximity.[4]

THE PROCEDURES INVOLVING THE UTEROSACRAL LIGAMENT

Prophylactic Suspension in Hysterectomy

Given that the USL is a primary support structure for the uterus, it is standard practice to anchor vaginal vault with the distal segment of the USL during hysterectomy. This helps in preventing vault prolapse in future.

Fothergill Hysteropexy

In this technique, the cardinal ligament complex (Mackenrodt's and USL) is severed from its attachment to cervix and repositioned them on cervix

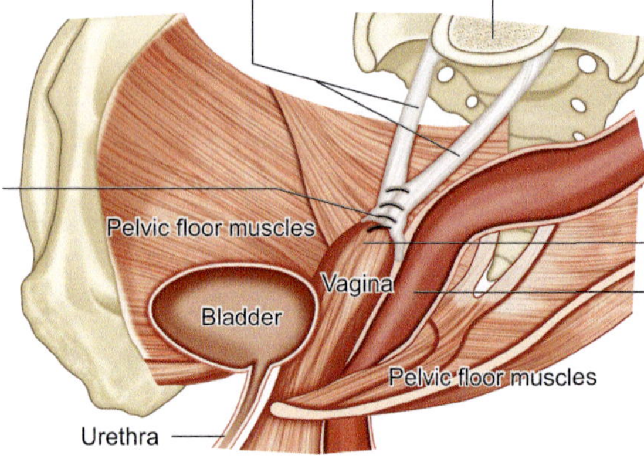

Fig. 6: In-vault descent noticed during hysterectomies.

on midline anteriorly. This causes shortening of ligaments and elevates the uterus effectively while maintaining anteflexion and anteversion.

McCall's Culdoplasty

This procedure involves two key components and involves the lower segment of the USL:

1. USLs are approximated in the midline thereby reducing the length virtually and obliterating the lax pouch of Douglas—internal McCall sutures.
2. The vault is elevated by securing it to both USLs, proximal to the previous sutures, referred to as external McCall sutures.

This approach is particularly beneficial in less severe degree of prolapse, and also in vault descent noticed during hysterectomies **(Fig. 6)**.

HIGH UTEROSACRAL LIGAMENT SUSPENSION PROCEDURE[5]

In this technique, the intermediate segment of USL is taken as the suspension point to fix and support the prolapsed structures. This point is determined on the basis on the available vaginal length to ensure a tension-free repair. Excessive tension at the suspension point may lead to avulsion and failure of the procedure **(Fig. 7)**.

Multiple sutures are threaded through the USL and their free ends are passed through the angle of the vault.

In case of hysteropexy, the sutures are passed through the ligament complex attached to the cervix laterally. While tying these sutures, the vault gets lifted up to the sacral hollow.

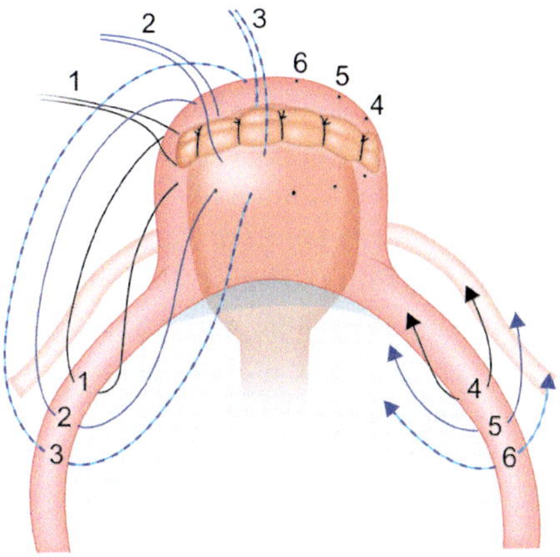

Fig. 7: Principles of high uterosacral ligament suspension. Series of suture pass—from mid USL (1, 2, 3 of patient's left side and 4, 5, 6 of right side) to vault to recreate the dome of vaginal apex.

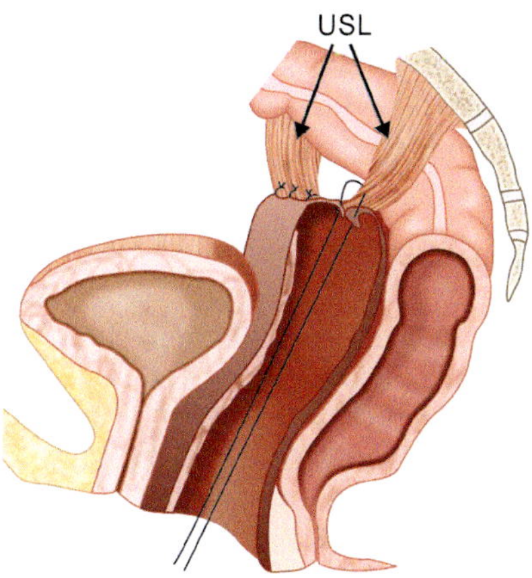

Fig. 8: Position of vagina following high uterosacral ligament suspension.

This procedure is bilateral in nature, suspends angle of the vault to the ipsilateral USL. As a result, the vaginal canal maintains its normal anatomy, including length, caliber, curvature, and axis, while preserving the soft and suppleness of birth canal **(Fig. 8)**.

Drawbacks of Procedures Involving the Uterosacral Ligament

The ureter runs parallel and in close proximity to the USL inside the pelvis, leading to high chances of ureteric complications. These complications are in the form of kinking, direct injury, and complete or partial blockage, which may not be evident intraoperative. To minimize these risks, intraoperative cystoscopy is recommended to detect complications as they arise so that the necessary steps can be taken to avoid morbidity.

Theoretically, procedures involving the lower segment of the USL-like prophylactic suspension during hysterectomies and McCall's culdoplasty, could present a higher incidence of ureteric complications compared to high uterosacral ligament suspension (HUSLS). However, because the cervical portion of the USL is more accessible and can be clearly visualized and palpated by surgeons, the incidence of complications tends to be lower in these cases compared to high suspensions.

CONCLUSION

As native tissue, USL is considered to be the best reliable option for suspension procedure in pelvic organ prolapse. The procedure maintains the vagina in its normal anatomical position. Both abdominal and vaginal routes can be opted for this type of procedure with equal results. The role of laparoscopy is definitely of great advantage in visualizing these structures and keeping the ureter in safe zone. Care should be taken to confirm the ureteral patency during the surgery, for which intraoperative check cystoscopy is highly recommended. With experience and skill, expertise can be gained to make this Novel procedure safe and patient friendly.

REFERENCES

1. Jenkins VR 2nd. Uterosacral ligament fixation for vaginal vault suspension in uterine and vaginal vault prolapse. Am J Obstet Gynecol. 1997;177(6):1337-43; discussion 1343-4. doi: 10.1016/s0002-9378(97)70073-5. PMID: 9423733.
2. Buller JL, Thompson JR, Cundiff GW, Krueger Sullivan L, Schön Ybarra MA, Bent AE. Uterosacral ligament: description of anatomic relationships to optimize surgical safety. Obstet Gynecol. 2001;97(6):873-9. doi: 10.1016/s0029-7844(01)01346-1. PMID: 11384688.
3. Kieserman-Shmokler C, Swenson CW, Chen L, Desmond LM, Ashton-Miller JA, DeLancey JO. From molecular to macro: the key role of the apical ligaments in uterovaginal support. Am J Obstet Gynecol. 2020;222(5):427-36. doi: 10.1016/j.ajog.2019.10.006. Epub 2019 Oct 19. PMID: 31639371; PMCID: PMC7166152.
4. Sajadi KP, Vasavada S. Uterosacral Ligament Suspension. In: Goldman H (Eds). Complications of Female Incontinence and Pelvic Reconstructive Surgery. Current Clinical Urology, 2017. Humana Press, Cham. https://doi.org/10.1007/978-3-319-49855-37.
5. Verma A, Kashyap M, Gupta A. High uterosacral ligament fixation versus McCall's culdoplasty for vaginal vault suspension in uterovaginal prolapse surgery. Cureus. 2022;14(7):e27368. doi: 10.7759/cureus.27368. PMID: 36046323; PMCID: PMC9417864.

18

CHAPTER

Role of Vessel Sealers in Vaginal Surgeries

Punam Dixit, Monika Anant

INTRODUCTION

Vessel sealing devices have revolutionized vaginal hysterectomy, enhancing the efficiency and safety of the procedure. Traditional methods, such as "clamp, cut, ligate," often present challenges in confined spaces and complex anatomical conditions. The introduction of electrobipolar vessel sealing technology, starting with Ligasure in 1998, has significantly improved surgical outcomes by providing precise hemostasis, reducing blood loss, and minimizing the need for manual suturing. These advancements offer numerous benefits, including shorter operative times, less postoperative pain, and quicker recovery. This technology has expanded the indications for vaginal hysterectomy, making it an increasingly preferred approach in gynecological surgery.

Vaginal hysterectomy is considered the gold standard in minimal access surgery, offering key benefits such as faster recovery, shorter hospital stays, reduced postoperative pain, and fewer complications. It has become the preferred approach over open abdominal and laparoscopic routes. Since the early innovations introduced by Kelly, the integration of newer technologies has significantly eased the procedure, helping surgeons overcome challenges like limited access and deep suturing. The introduction of Electrobipolar Vessel-Sealing Devices (EBVS) in 1998, beginning with LigaSure, revolutionized the field. Randomized controlled trials have since confirmed the safety and efficacy of these devices. Presently, multiple devices are available, some designed for single use while others are reusable. Reusable devices, in particular, offer a more cost-effective solution compared to their single-use counterparts, making them ideal for settings with financial constraints. These technological advancements continue to improve surgical outcomes, making vaginal hysterectomy safer and more efficient than ever.

The traditional *'clamp, cut, ligate'* method is the standard approach in vaginal hysterectomy, requiring sufficient vaginal space for instrument manipulation. This technique involves clamping, cutting, and ligating the uterine ligaments and vessels while ensuring hemostasis at each step.

Minimal hemostasis is typically required during the dissection of the anterior and posterior vaginal walls and when opening the vesicovaginal and recto-vaginal peritoneal folds. Instruments commonly used include hysterectomy clamps, tissue scissors, needle holders, artery forceps, and retractors to support the vaginal walls, facilitating a controlled and efficient surgical process.

However, space constraints can pose significant challenges in traditional vaginal hysterectomy methods, particularly in cases such as non-descent vaginal hysterectomy, uterine enlargement due to adenomyosis or fibroids, narrow subpubic angles, and the need for adnexectomy in deep pelvic regions. These factors can restrict instrument movement and limit exposure, complicating the surgical procedure. Advanced bipolar vessel-sealing instruments are particularly beneficial for women with limited vaginal access, such as those with a high body mass index, orthopedic conditions that restrict hip abduction, or a narrow pubic arch. These devices require less operative space than traditional clamps and suture ligation, making them an effective option in challenging anatomical situations.

This highlighted the need for instruments that could coagulate and achieve hemostasis at the vaginal stumps, eliminating the requirement for suturing. By the optimized combination of pressure and radiofrequency/ultrasonic energies, vessel sealers generate energy targeted to the tissue impedance, efficiently sealing blood vessels up to 7 mm diameter with risk of thermal injury limited to only 2 mm on the grasped tissue. Studies have shown that in vaginal hysterectomies for benign conditions, electrosurgical bipolar vessel-sealing devices have been compared to conventional clamping and suturing techniques. For vaginal hysterectomies using vessel-sealing devices, the outcomes of self-reported pain levels and quality-of-life were promising even after 6 months **(Fig. 1)**.

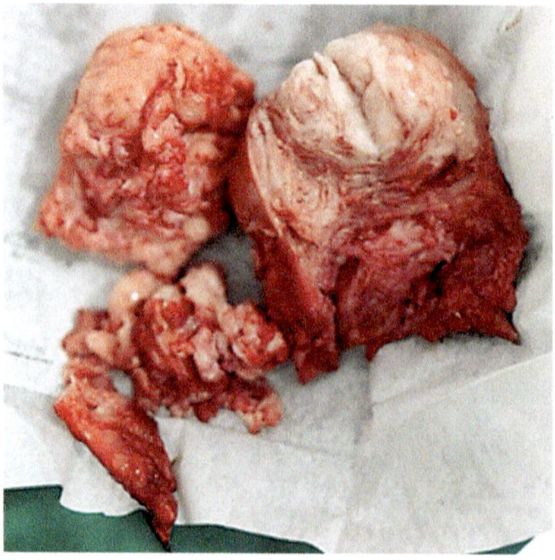

Fig. 1: 22-weeks' sized fibroid uterus specimen (weight 800 g) after vaginal hysterectomy with advanced vessel sealer.

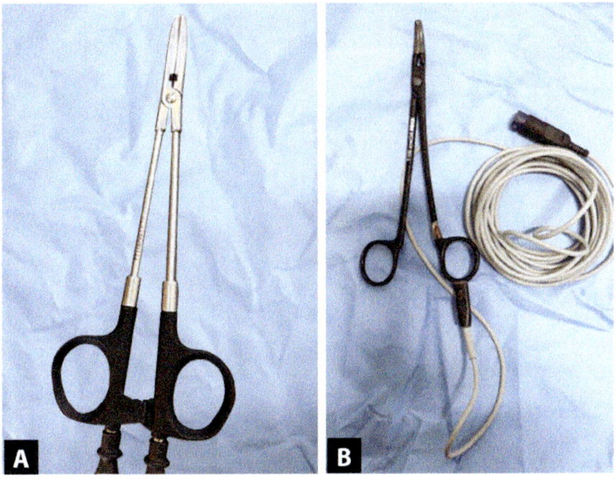

Figs. 2A and B: Vessel-sealing devices.

If the adnexa cannot be easily removed using standard techniques, laparoscopic or handheld electrosurgical vessel-sealing devices are often employed transvaginally to facilitate effective removal **(Figs. 2A and B)**. These tools enhance precision and control, allowing surgeons to navigate challenging anatomical conditions during the procedure.

Many gynecological oncologists have identified standard vaginal hysterectomy (VH) as a viable alternative to other surgical approaches for endometrial cancer, particularly in patients with obesity, those over 65 years of age, or individuals with compromised surgical fitness due to medical conditions.

Bipolar vessel-sealing technology has significantly improved surgical outcomes in vaginal hysterectomies by offering a more efficient and less invasive alternative to the traditional "clamp, cut, ligate" method.

Several advantages make this approach particularly appealing:

Enhanced efficiency of the surgical steps leads to reduced operative time: Bipolar vessel-sealing devices work by applying precise energy to seal vessels and tissues, providing hemostasis almost instantaneously. This eliminates the need for manual suturing at the vaginal stumps, which traditionally requires time-consuming manipulation of clamps, sutures, and needle holders in limited space. By removing these manual steps, surgeons can reduce overall operative time, which not only increases efficiency but also minimizes the patient's exposure to anesthesia.

Improved hemostasis by these instruments leads to reduced overall blood loss by its ability to achieve consistent and reliable hemostasis. The device applies controlled energy that causes protein denaturation within the tissue, leading to a permanent seal of vessels up to 7 mm in diameter. In comparison, traditional suturing can sometimes lead to suboptimal hemostasis,

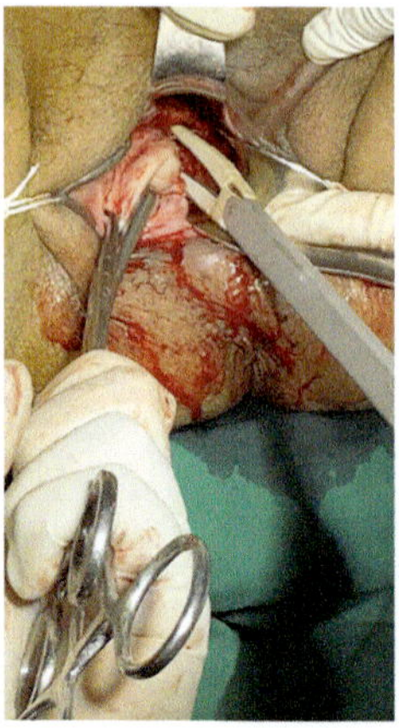

Fig. 3: Coagulation of uterine artery.

particularly in cases with anatomical challenges such as non-descent hysterectomy or uterine enlargement due to fibroids or adenomyosis **(Fig. 3)**. It is a significant advantage as it decreases the chances of postoperative complications and the need for postoperative blood transfusions.

Minimum tissue handling leads to *minimized tissue trauma* while traditional suturing techniques require more tissue manipulation, more so in areas where exposure is limited or difficult, such as the vaginal vault or narrow subpubic angles. Excessive tissue handling may result in inflammation, edema, or tissue damage, prolonging recovery. Bipolar vessel-sealing minimizes tissue trauma by applying targeted energy only where needed, preserving surrounding tissues and facilitating faster healing.

It has been found to *reduce postoperative pain* and lead to *faster recovery* and shorter hospital stays. In studies where patients were blinded to the surgical technique used, those who underwent procedures with vessel-sealing technology reported less pain and quicker return to daily activities compared to those who underwent traditional suturing.

Decreased risk of complications such as postoperative hemorrhage, infections, and wound dehiscence are seen when bipolar vessel sealing is employed. The risk of suture-related complications, such as granulomas or tissue irritation, is also eliminated.

Because of its relative ease of use it is more easy to adopt vessel-sealing methods, *learning curve is short*. A significant advantage of bipolar vessel sealing is its relative ease of use. Surgeons and residents who may have limited experience with traditional suturing techniques in vaginal hysterectomy settings can easily adapt to this technique.

Many raise the concern of the cost of instruments, while the upfront costs of bipolar vessel-sealing devices may be higher than traditional instruments,

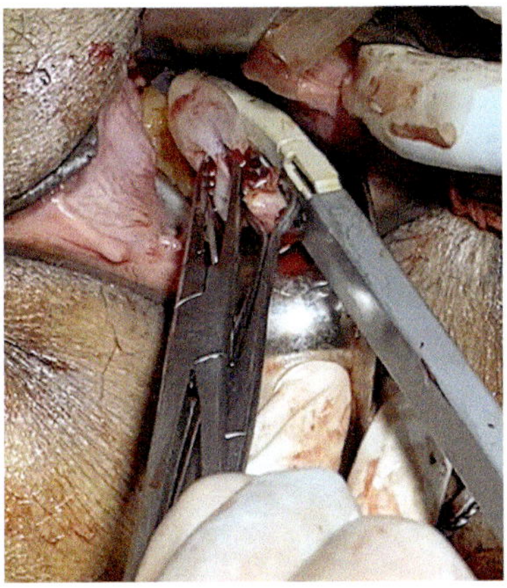

Fig. 4: Salpingectomy.

the overall cost-effectiveness becomes apparent when considering the reduced operative time, lesser sutures used, lower complication rates, and shorter hospital stays. Moreover, the potential for reduced blood transfusions, reoperation, or interventions further justifies the investment in advanced vessel-sealing technology.

PRECAUTIONS AND PRACTICAL TIPS

Working in a confined vaginal space can pose a risk of thermal injury to nearby organs—such as the bladder, ureters, or rectum. Thermal spread is limited to less than 1.5-2.00 mm beyond the grasped tissues. However, adjacent structures should be protected by adequate exposure with suitable retractors. The tip of the instrument should not be in contact with wet sponges or fluid to avoid injury to other organs. Surgeons must be vigilant to avoid thermal spread and unintended damage **(Fig. 4)**.

The pedicles to be coagulated should not be under tension and very broad. If pedicles are large, taking all at one go is not wide, smaller width of pedicles can be coagulated at multiple times to achieve complete seal. Although vessel sealers are recommended to coagulate vessels up to 7 mm caliber, with larger uteruses like fibroids or adenomyosis >12 weeks may have vessels of larger caliber where additional suturing will be required to secure the pedicle.

In cases of adnexectomy, while securing the infundibulopelvic ligament our practice is to clamp and then coagulate to avoid the slippage of pedicles **(Fig. 5)**. After ensuring complete coagulation the pedicle should be irrigated with normal saline to check for complete hemostasis and cool off the surrounding tissue. This also prevents any inadvertent injury to other organs.

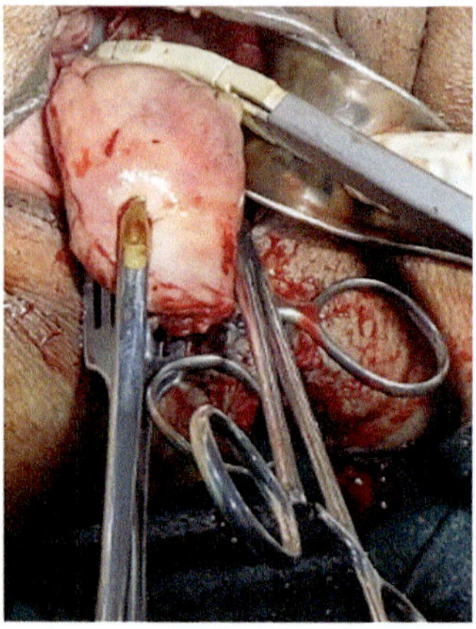

Fig. 5: Coagulation of infundibulopelvic ligament.

By personal experience of authors, it has been observed that the texture of the tissue and pedicles can be very soft and fragile if the women are on progesterone therapy for abnormal uterine bleeding (AUB) for a long time. This requires much gentler tissue handling and suturing can sometimes cut through the pedicles, whereas vessel sealers are of use here to achieve complete and safe hemostasis.

Bipolar vessel-sealing devices have thus transformed the landscape of vaginal surgery by offering numerous benefits. The few limitations to consider are cost as they are more expensive than traditional surgical tools like clamps, scissors, and sutures. Upfront costs maybe high but overall cost effectiveness by reducing other costs balances such investments and can prove profitable.

All devices are susceptible to malfunction, so relying solely on a single instrument can be counterproductive. However, with advanced features, such failures are rare, but surgeons must still be prepared to revert to traditional methods when necessary.

Proper training and expertise in the use of vessel-sealing devices are crucial for residents to achieve optimal results. Surgeons must be well-versed in the device's energy settings, application techniques, and safety precautions.

Vessel-sealing devices may have limited utility in complex cases involving extensive adhesions or distorted anatomy, such as those resulting from previous surgeries, endometriosis, or severe pelvic inflammatory disease. In such scenarios, traditional techniques often offer better control and flexibility. Manual suturing or ligation may be preferred due to the need for more precise tissue handling and dissection. However, some reports suggest that vessel-sealing devices can still provide notable benefits, particularly in challenging procedures. The balance between traditional and advanced methods remains essential for optimal outcomes.

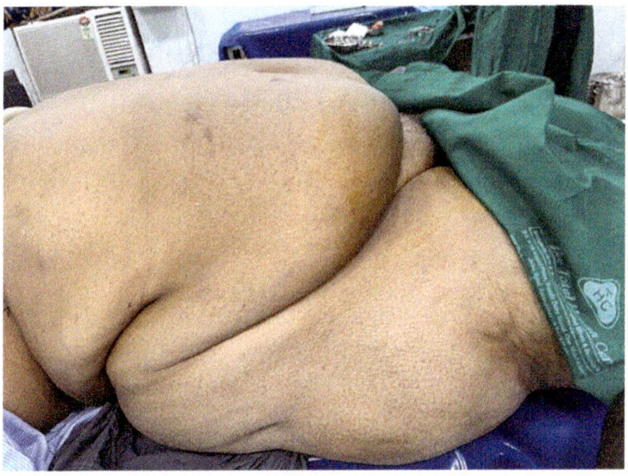

Fig. 6: Vaginal hysterectomy bilateral salpingo-oophorectomy for 120 kg patient.

The reliance on advanced technology and a stable power supply may limit the device's functionality in resource-constrained settings. In environments with inconsistent electricity or infrastructure, its usability could be significantly reduced.

Less experienced surgeons may develop an overreliance on bipolar vessel-sealing devices, leading to potential overuse in surgical practice **(Fig. 6)**. This dependency can hinder the development of essential suturing skills, particularly among younger surgeons who may not gain adequate experience with traditional techniques. As a result, the proficiency in fundamental surgical methods could decline over time.

The indications and complexity for vaginal hysterectomy have broadened to include cases previously deemed unsuitable for this approach, thanks to the introduction of vessel-sealing systems. These advancements, supported by evidence of safety, efficacy, and improved patient outcomes, have expanded the scope of vaginal surgeries.

CONCLUSION

Bipolar vessel-sealing technology represents a significant advancement in vaginal surgery, particularly for hysterectomy procedures. The benefits of reduced operative time, improved hemostasis, lower complication rates, and faster recovery make it a superior alternative to traditional suturing methods. As more gynecologists gain experience with these devices, bipolar vessel sealing is likely to become standard practice, particularly in cases where space constraints and complex anatomical conditions present surgical challenges.

Despite their many advantages, bipolar vessel-sealing devices come with certain drawbacks, such as higher costs, the potential for device malfunction, and a risk of thermal injury. Additionally, they may not be suitable for all surgical cases, especially those involving complex anatomy or extensive adhesions. Surgeons need to balance the benefits of using these devices with limitations, ensuring they are properly trained and have a clear understanding of when to use vessel-sealing versus traditional methods.

While other technologies noted in the literature show promise for enhancing vaginal surgical procedures and improving outcomes, further comparative effectiveness research is necessary to validate these benefits.

SUGGESTED READING

1. Bentham GL, Preshaw J. Review of advanced energy devices for the minimal access gynaecologist. The Obstetrician & Gynaecologist. 2021;23:301-9. doi:10.1111/tog.12774.
2. Dubey P, Dube M, Kanhere A, Biswas N, De R, Koley A, Banerjee PK. Electrothermal vessel sealing versus conventional suturing in abdominal hysterectomy: a randomised trial. Cureus. 2023;15(1):e34123. doi: 10.7759/cureus.34123. PMID: 36843794; PMCID: PMC9947513.
3. Ellaithy M, Agur W. The advantages in the selection and use of vessel sealing devices in vaginal hysterectomy, dependent on the different degrees of operative difficulty. Springer International Publishing, Switzwerland. 2018. pp. 1443-55.
4. Haughey N, Beirne JP, Blayney GV, Hinds L, Quinn D, Chandranath D, Dorman GJ. Vaginal hysterecto™y using the ERBE BiClamp® bipolar vessel sealing system as a surgical approach for endometrial cancer: single surgeon experience from a district general hospital. Eur J Gynaecol Oncol. 2022;43(6):26-33.
5. Hefni MA, Bhaumik J, El-Touky T, Kho P, Wong I, Abdel-Razik T, et al. Safety and efficacy of using LigaSure vessel sealing system for securing the pedicles in vaginal hysterectomy: randomized controlled trial. BJOG. 2005;112(3):329-33.

19

CHAPTER

Is Hysterectomy a Necessary Component of a Surgery for Prolapse?

Pankaj Sarode

INTRODUCTION

India, home to 1.4 billion people, has surpassed mainland China to become the world's most populous country, according to UN estimates. This gives India potential advantage of a demographic dividend. India has about 65% population in the age group of 15–60 years. Although it is a huge advantage for India to fulfill its economic growth, it rings an alarm that we will have a large number of populations above 60 years of age by 2050. According to one estimate India will have a population of 35 crores above the age of 60 by 2050. By present statistics, pelvic organ prolapse affects about 40% women above the age of 50.11% of whom would need one or more surgeries for the prolapse in their lifetime. Recurrence risk of 30% is significantly high for any mode of presently available surgeries for POP. Hence, surgeries for POP need re-evaluation and modifications to decrease risk of recurrence and to improve results in terms of postsurgery quality of life for women.

The efficacy and safety of removing or preserving the uterus during reconstructive pelvic surgery is debatable. Techniques that include subtotal or total hysterectomy are the most common approaches to the repair of symptomatic uterine prolapse. However, some authors consider that hysterectomy increases the risk of complications and morbidity and question the need for uterine removal, while others believe that prolapse will recur more frequently if the uterus is preserved.

It has been a dictum to perform hysterectomy and vaginal wall repairs for complaints of prolapse, so far. Since we know that the uterus is not the cause of prolapse but a 'casualty' of the injury sustained to the pelvic floor. With changing lifestyle, we are getting more and more women asking for uterus preservation surgeries. As women have started planning pregnancies later in life and with easy accessibility to egg-freezing—ART services, a few of them may be interested in preserving their fertility potential as well. Also are into consideration sexual effects of uterus removal surgeries which were not as important as they are in present era. So, it is worth asking ourselves about need for uterus removal for complaints of prolapse. Especially for cases with lower grades of anatomical deficiencies.

An article published in International Urogynecological Association's Journal which is about a meta-analysis of studies comparing utero-preservation to uterus removal concludes following points:

RECURRENCE RATE

Recurrence rate was defined as recurrence of symptoms by the woman. Data of about 400 patients in each group, hystero-preservation and hysterectomy with suspension, were compared. The overall conclusion was that the recurrence rate was lower for hysterectomy as compared to hysteropexy. While analyzing cases depending upon surgical procedures and approaches (abdominal, vaginal, or laparoscopic), it was found that for vaginal route recurrence was lower for hysterectomy with native tissue repair than for hystero-preservation procedures. It is interesting to note that recurrences were less for vaginal hysterectomy with native tissue repairs as compared to abdominal sacro-colpopexy even when the mesh was used to reinforce uterosacral ligaments for abdominal procedures.

REOPERATION RATES

Reoperation rate was lower with vaginal hysterectomy with repairs than for hysteropexy for all routes, abdominal or vaginal. Vaginal hysterectomy with Sacro-spinous ligament fixation had lower reoperation rate (2.4%) as compared to abdominal sacro-colpopexy (22%) in one study.

The secondary outcomes like operative time and blood loss, as expected, were less with hystero-preservation. The rates of visceral injuries were the same for both the groups.

VOIDING DYSFUNCTION

Although analyses have shown no differences in the rates of voiding dysfunctions following procedures preserving and removing the uterus, it was observed that the rate was lower following hysteropexy via the vaginal route. Dietz et al. observed voiding dysfunction rates of 8.5% (3 of 35 patients) with vaginal hysteropexy and 25.8% (8 of 31 patients) with vaginal hysterectomy, both with sacrospinous fixation with native tissue. On the other hand, for procedures performed via the abdominal route, the rate of voiding dysfunction tended to be lower with hysterectomy. Costantini et al. reported voiding dysfunction rates of 11.8 and 2.6% for abdominal hystero-sacropexy and abdominal hysterectomy with colpo-sacropexy, respectively.

Duration of Hospitalization

There was no significant difference in the length of hospital stay for both the groups.

Mesh Exposure

Although meshes are not in use at present for prolapse repair. The available data from the studies when meshes were used showed higher incidence after hysterectomy for vaginal as well as abdominal approach as compared to hystero-preservation.

Dyspareunia

There was no significant difference. All routes and all techniques had the same incidence of dyspareunia meaning no technique had an advantage above others when taking sexual satisfaction into consideration.[1]

CONCLUSION

With increasing depth of knowledge about surgical anatomy of pelvis and with evolution of surgical techniques, it is imperative to question the need for a radical approach like hysterectomy for repair of symptoms of prolapse. Although present knowledge based on available studies acknowledge the advantage of traditional techniques of vaginal hysterectomy with native tissue repair one needs to understand that the inherent recurrence rate for this procedure is disheartening. The sparsely available studies using vaginal mesh favor its use, presently available meshes are not suitable for vaginal use due to high rates of mesh erosion. Research into ideal mesh material for vaginal use is bound to succeed and the future holds huge potential for use of meshes for prolapse repair. Even if the recurrence rates are similar with lesser operative time and lesser blood loss, hystero-preservation procedures can be used for selected few patients with perioperative risks due to morbidities. Also, women present with different components of apical and vaginal wall prolapse. A few of them without much apical component may be an ideal candidates for uterus preservation surgeries.[2]

Women would prefer not to remove uterus if it is not absolutely necessary. So, till we have an option with minimal recurrence and reoperation risk, we should keep on revisiting this question—to remove or not to remove the uterus for prolapse.[3]

REFERENCES

1. de Oliveira SA, Fonseca MCM, Bortolini MAT, Girão MJBC, Roque MT, Castro RA. Hystero-preservation versus hysterectomy in the surgical treatment of uterine prolapse: systematic review and meta-analysis. Int Urogynecol J. 2017;28:1617-30.
2. Costantini E, Mearini L, Bini V, Zucchi A, Mearini E, Porena M. Uterus preservation in surgical correction of urogenital prolapse. Eur Urol. 2005;48:642-9.
3. Dietz V, van der Vaart CH, van der Graaf Y, Heintz P, Koops SES. One-year follow-up after sacrospinous hysteropexy and vaginal hysterectomy for uterine descensus: a randomized study. Int Urogynecol J. 2010;21:209-16.

20 CHAPTER

Complications of Vaginal Surgeries

Nilakshi Phukan Kumar

INTRODUCTION

Vaginal surgery encompasses a wide range of procedures, including hysterectomy, vaginoplasty, and labiaplasty, which are performed to address various medical conditions and enhance quality of life. While these surgeries offer numerous benefits, they also carry inherent risks and potential complications. This article provides a comprehensive overview of the complications associated with vaginal surgery, drawing from multiple peer-reviewed sources and expert opinions **(Fig. 1)**.

GENERAL RISKS AND COMPLICATIONS

As with any surgical procedure, vaginal surgery carries general risks that patients and healthcare providers must be aware of:

Anesthetic Complications

Although rare, anesthetic accidents in the form of allergic reaction to respiratory and cardiovascular issues can occur during vaginal surgery.[1]

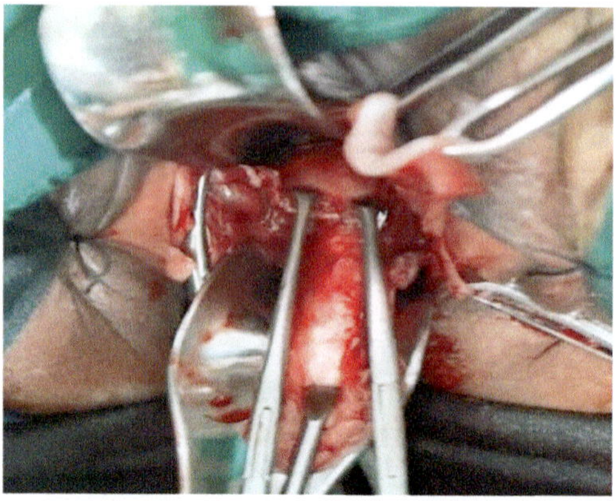

Fig. 1: Vaginal surgery encompasses.

Intraoperative Complications

Bleeding

Hemorrhage remains a primary concern during vaginal surgeries. The most common sites of bleeding during vaginal hysterectomy are uterine vessels, utero-ovarian ligament, and vaginal cuff.[2] Incidence of intraoperative heavy bleeding is about 1–5%.[3]

Injection of adrenaline diluted with normal saline or normal saline alone into the vaginal wall not only reduces the blood loss but also facilitates the dissection of vaginal wall. Uterine vessels must be ligated properly including both reflected peritoneal margins. Uses of newer vessel-sealing devices reduce intraoperative bleeding.

Urinary Tract Injuries

Ureteral injury: The incidence of ureteral injury is about 0.05–0.1%.[3]

Ureteric injuries mostly occur at the following sites: Clamping and cutting of infundibulopelvic ligaments, dissecting the uterine artery and during the closure of vaginal vault **(Figs. 2A and B)**.[4]

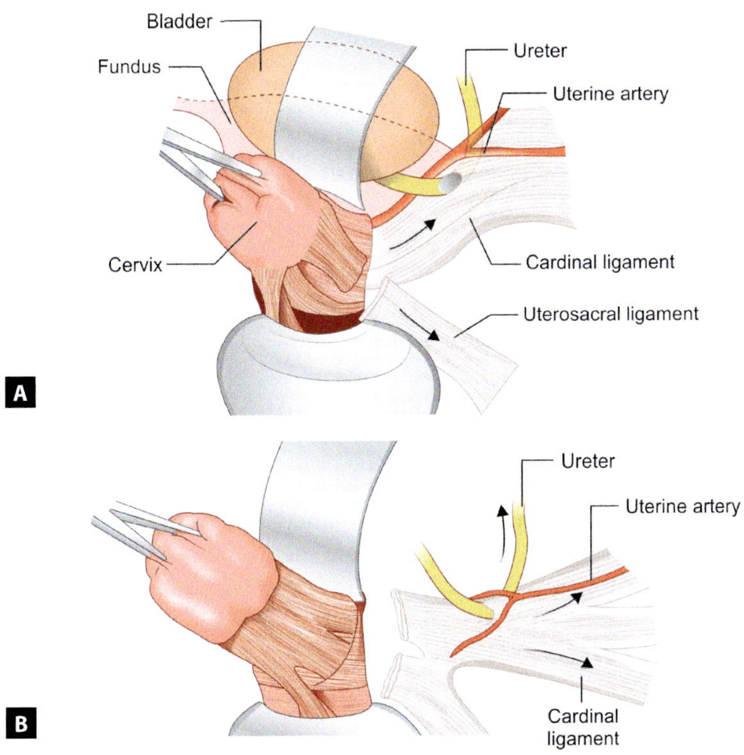

Figs. 2A and B: Ureter and uterine artery.

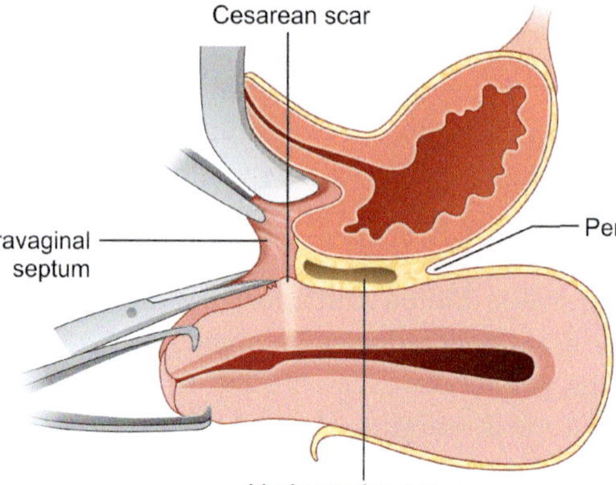

Fig. 3: Urinary bladder injury.

Urinary bladder injury: The prevalence of bladder injury during vaginal hysterectomy varies between 0.5–1.5%.[3] Chance of injury is more in patients with prior pelvic surgeries and cesarean section. Most common time of bladder injury is during entry into the anterior cul-de-sac **(Fig. 3)**.[5]

To minimize urinary tract injuries:
- Sharp dissection rather than blunt tearing of tissues avoids distortion of anatomic planes
- Consider backfilling the bladder for better visualization
- Traction on a uterine manipulator
- Perform intraoperative cystoscopy when indicated

Bowel Injury

Although less common than urinary tract injuries, bowel perforation can occur during vaginal surgery, particularly in cases with extensive adhesions or during complex pelvic reconstructive procedures.

CONVERSION TO LAPAROTOMY

Instances like unexpected large pelvic masses, adhesions, and hemorrhage unable to identify and control can increase the chances of conversion to abdominal hysterectomy. Preoperative assessment of patients is very much essential preferably under anesthesia to see the mobility. Use of various electrosurgical instruments can minimize the risk of hemorrhage.

POSTOPERATIVE COMPLICATIONS

Infections

One of the most common complications associated with vaginal surgery is infection. The vaginal canal hosts a diverse microbial environment, and any disruption due to surgery can predispose individuals to bacterial, fungal, or viral infections. There are wide variations of incidence 0.2–10%.[3]

Urinary tract infection is the most frequent postoperative complication following vaginal surgeries. Recent studies have reported UTI rates of 11.8% within 8 weeks post-hysterectomy, with higher rates (21.7%) observed in cases combining hysterectomy with pelvic reconstructive surgery.[6] Risk factors for posthysterectomy UTIs include:

- Premenopausal status
- Anterior vaginal wall prolapse
- Postvoid residual urine >150 mL
- Long operative time
- Adhesiolysis during surgery
- Ileus development[7,8]

Proper preoperative preparation, perioperative antibiotic prophylaxis, and meticulous surgical techniques are essential in mitigating these risks.

Urinary Dysfunctions

Vaginal surgery can inadvertently affect the adjacent urinary structures, leading to urinary retention and incontinence. Bladder injury or disruption of pelvic floor muscle can contribute to these complications. Incidence of postoperative VVF is about 0.1–0.2%.[3]

Postoperative Vault Prolapse

Incidence of postoperative prolapse is more when the surgery is performed for genital organ prolapse (RCOG Green Top Guidelines 46).

A recent 10-year follow-up study reported that 1.6% of women who underwent hysterectomy for benign indications subsequently required POP surgery. Risk factors for post-hysterectomy POP include:

- History of vaginal deliveries **(Fig. 4)**
- Concomitant stress urinary incontinence surgery[8]

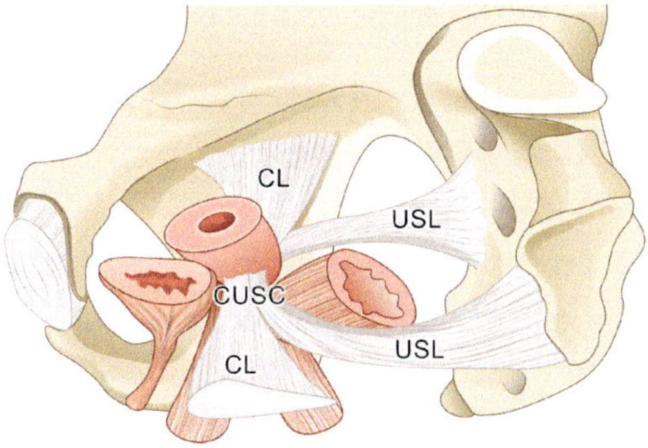

Fig. 4: Vault suspension. (CL: cardinal ligament; CUSC: cardinal uterosacral complex; USL: uterosacral ligament)

To prevent POP the following steps to be considered:

- Attaching uterosacral ligament and the cardinal ligament to the vaginal membrane
- Closure of the cul-de-sac

Position-related Complications

As vaginal surgery is done in lithotomy position, patients are at risk for developing some specific complications.

Lower Extremities Neuropathies

Prolonged pressure on nerves, particularly the peroneal nerve, can result in temporary or, rarely, permanent nerve damage. Symptoms may include numbness, tingling, or weakness in the affected limb.[9]

Acute compartment syndrome (ACS)—though infrequent may occur due to lithotomy position.[1,9] ACS is seen particularly after prolonged surgery lasting beyond 2–4 hours.[10,11] Delayed diagnosis may lead to irreversible muscle necrosis and even requiring delayed lower limb amputation.[12,13]

To prevent positioning-related complications include:

- Careful patient positioning with adequate padding
- Regular repositioning during prolonged procedures
- Monitoring of extremities during and immediately after surgery
- Early mobilization in the postoperative period

Sexual Dysfunction

Complications in the form of bleeding, stenosis, injury to the other viscera including fistulas and scarring may occur during surgery and in postoperative periods. There may be postoperative sexual dysfunction after vaginoplasty and labioplasty. There are changes in sensation, lubrication or aesthetic appearance after surgery. These may impact sexual satisfaction and psychological wellbeing. Discussion with the patient prior to surgery is very essential.

COMPLICATIONS OF VAGINAL RECONSTRUCTIVE SURGERIES

Complications Specific to Vaginoplasty

Vaginoplasty, a procedure often performed as part of gender affirmation surgery, carries its own set of complications:

- *Neovaginal stenosis:* Regular dilation is crucial to maintain vaginal depth and width.[7] Adherence to the dilation regimen for at least one-year postoperatively is beneficial.

- *Granulation tissue:* The formation of granulation tissue in the neovagina is common and can lead to discharge and discomfort. Treatment with silver nitrate, topical steroids, or medical-grade honey for persistent cases are beneficial.
- *Neovaginal prolapse:* Although rare, prolapse of the neovagina can occur and may require surgical correction.
- *Rectovaginal fistula:* This serious complication can result from injury to the rectum during surgery. These fistulas usually occur within 5 cm of the vaginal opening and may require a temporary diverting colostomy for management.

Complications of Vaginal Rejuvenation Procedures

Vaginal rejuvenation procedures, such as labiaplasty and vulvoplasty, carry their own set of risks:

- *Asymmetry:* Uneven healing or tissue removal can result in asymmetrical appearance of the labia or vulva.
- *Overcorrection:* Excessive tissue removal can lead to functional problems or dissatisfaction with the aesthetic outcome.
- *Chronic pain:* Some patients may experience long-term pain or discomfort in the treated area.
- *Sexual dysfunction:* Changes in sensation or appearance may impact sexual satisfaction and psychological well-being.

To Minimize the Risk of Complications in Vaginal Surgery

- Careful preoperative assessment and patient selection are crucial.
- Meticulous surgical technique and adherence to best practices can significantly reduce the risk of complications.
- Close monitoring and appropriate postoperative care are essential for early detection and management of complications.
- Thorough preoperative counselling and clear postoperative instructions can help patients recognize and report potential complications early.

CONCLUSION

Vaginal surgery, while offering significant benefits in treating various gynecological conditions and enhancing quality of life, carries inherent risks and potential complications. By understanding these risks, implementing appropriate preventive measures, and providing comprehensive patient care, healthcare providers can optimize outcomes and patient satisfaction. As surgical techniques continue to evolve, ongoing research and vigilant monitoring of complications will be crucial in further improving the safety and efficacy of vaginal surgical procedures.

REFERENCES

1. Flierl MA, et al. Traction table-related complications in orthopaedic surgery. J Am Acad Orthop Surg. 2010;18(11):668-75. doi: 10.5435/00124635-201011000-00004.
2. Wood C, Maher P, Hill D. Bleeding associated with vaginal hysterectomy. Aust NZJ Obstet Gynaecol. 1997;37(4):457-61.
3. Te Linde's Operative Gynaecology, 11th edition. 2014. pp. 712.
4. Sorinola O, Begum R. Prevention and management of ureteric injuries. Hosp Med. 2005;66(6):329-34.
5. Gilmour DT, Das S, Flowerdew G. Rates of urinary tract injury from gynecologic surgery and the role of intraoperative cystoscopy. Obstet Gynecol. 2006;107(6):1366-72.
6. El-Nashar SA, et al. Obstet Gynecol. 2018;132(6):1347-57.
7. Meltzer T. Vaginoplasty procedures, complications, and aftercare. UCSF Transgender Care and Treatment Guidelines, Department of Family and Community Medicine, University of California San Francisco, 2016.
8. Kuittinen T, et al. Acta Obstet Gynecol Scand. 2023;102(5):556-66.
9. Hsu KL, et al The dangers of hemilithotomy positioning on traction tables: case report of a well-leg drop foot after contralateral femoral nailing. Patient Saf Surg. 2015;9:18. doi: 10.1186/s13037-015-0069-2.
10. Bauer EC, et al. Survey of compartment syndrome of the lower extremity after gynecological operations. Langenbecks Arch Surg. 2014;399(3):343-8. doi: 10.1007/s00423-014-1172-z.
11. Kikuchi T, Maeda H. Two cases of compartment syndrome of the lower extremities during surgery for gynecological malignancies. J Anesth. 2016;30:481-5. doi: 10.1007/s00540-015-2135-4.
12. Kent T, et al. Skin grafts provide durable end-bearing coverage for lower-extremity amputations with critical soft tissue loss. Orthopedics. 2013;36(2):132-5. doi: 10.3928/01477447-20130122-07.7.
13. Abdul W, et al. Lower extremity compartment syndrome in the setting of iliofemoral deep vein thrombosis, phlegmasia cerulea dolens and factor VII deficiency. BMJ Case Rep. 2016;2016:bcr2016215078.

21 CHAPTER

Postoperative Care in Vaginal Surgery: Ensuring a Smooth Recovery

Kanchan Sharma

INTRODUCTION

Vaginal surgical procedures such as hysterectomies, vaginal repairs, and vaginal reconstructions require careful postoperative care to ensure a smooth and complication-free recovery. The postoperative period is critical, and proper care can significantly impact the patient's overall health and well-being.[9]

WHAT IS POSTOPERATIVE CARE?

Postoperative period begins from the time the patient leaves operation room and ends with the follow-up visits by the surgeon. Postoperative care is given to patients after an operation, in order to minimize postoperative complications.[1] It is done for early detection and treatment of postoperative complications. Postoperative care is provided by:

- Post-anesthesia care unit (PACU)
- Surgical intensive care unit (SICU)

Immediate Postoperative Care (0–24 hours)

Immediate Postoperative Care and Assessment Need **(Figs. 1 and 2)**

- Vital signs/pain assessment
- Body system assessment
- Fluid and electrolyte balance
- *Surgical wound and dressing:*
    - Reinforce for first 24 hours
    - Circle the drainage and write date and time[2]
- Check drainage tubing
- Postoperative orders
- Side rails up should be there
- Call light in reach

During this time, pay attention to the following points:

- *Monitoring:* Close monitoring of vital signs, including blood pressure, pulse, and oxygen saturation **(Fig. 3)**.[3]

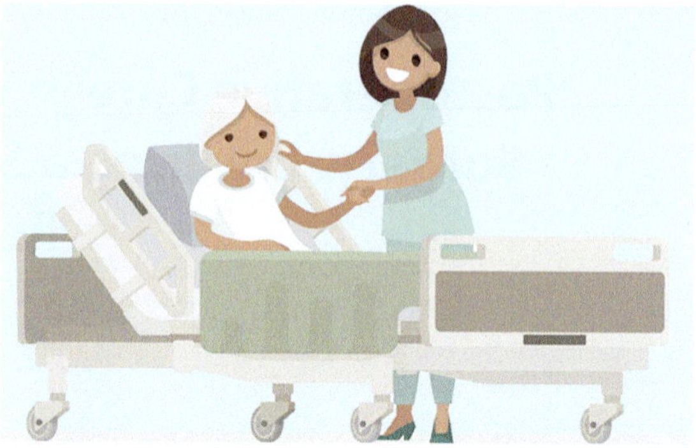

Fig. 1: Types and benefits of postoperative care.

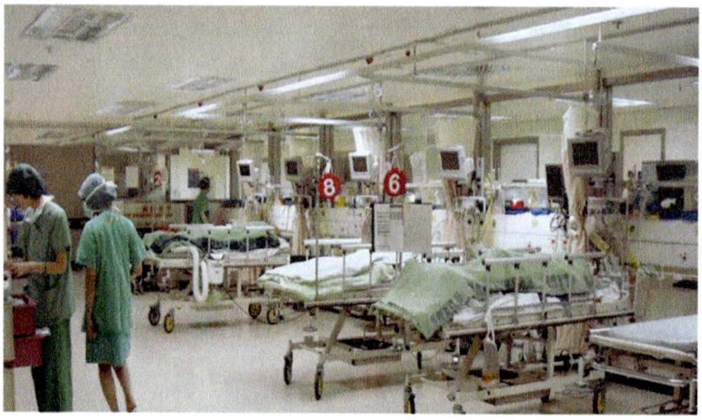

Fig. 2: Postoperative care.

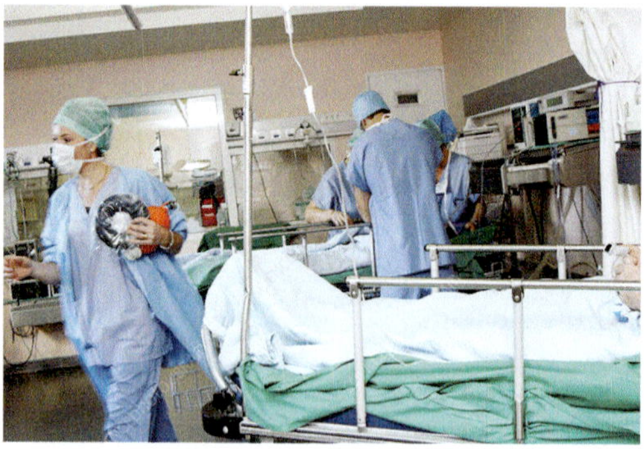

Fig. 3: Postoperative care system.

- *Pain management:* Effective pain management using analgesics and other pain relief methods.
- *Rest:* Complete bed rest for the first 24 hours to reduce bleeding and promote healing.
- *Hydration:* Encourage oral fluids to prevent dehydration.[4]

- *Urinary catheter:* A urinary catheter may be inserted to prevent urinary retention and promote healing.

Short-term Postoperative Care (24–72 hours)

- *Wound care:* It is necessary advice to keep the surgical site clean and dry to prevent infection.[5]
- *Dressing:* Utmost care to change dressings as directed by the healthcare provider.
- Pain management is to be looked postoperatively.
- Use postoperative laxative to prevent ileus[6]
- Mobility should be increased gradually to prevent blood clots and promote healing.
- *Diet:* Advised should be from liquids to solid foods as tolerated.

Long-term Postoperative Care (Beyond 72 hours)

- Follow-up appointments advice regarding it is very important.
- *Wound care:* Wound care and dressing changes as directed.[7]
- *Pelvic floor exercises:* Advise to begin pelvic floor exercises (Kegel exercises) to promote healing and prevent incontinence.[8]
- *Sexual activity:* Usually avoid sexual activity for 6–8 weeks after vaginal surgery, or as directed by the surgeon.
- *Heavy lifting:* For 6–8 weeks, avoid heavy lifting, bending, or strenuous activities[6]

Potential complications after the surgery, should be taken care of **(Fig. 4)**:

- *Infection:* Be attentive and monitor for signs of infection, such as fever, redness, or discharge.[10]

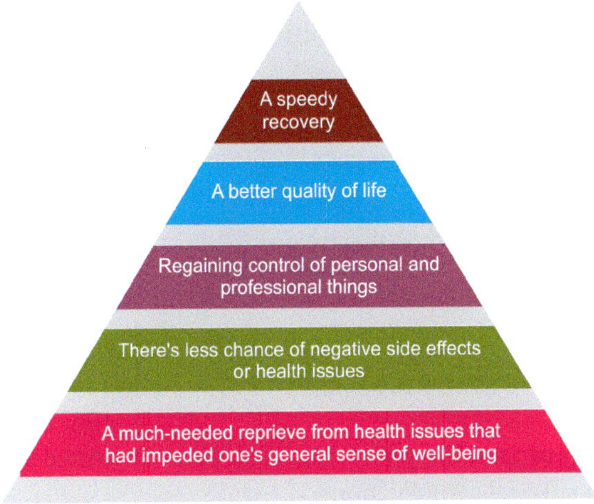

Fig. 4: Postoperative care.

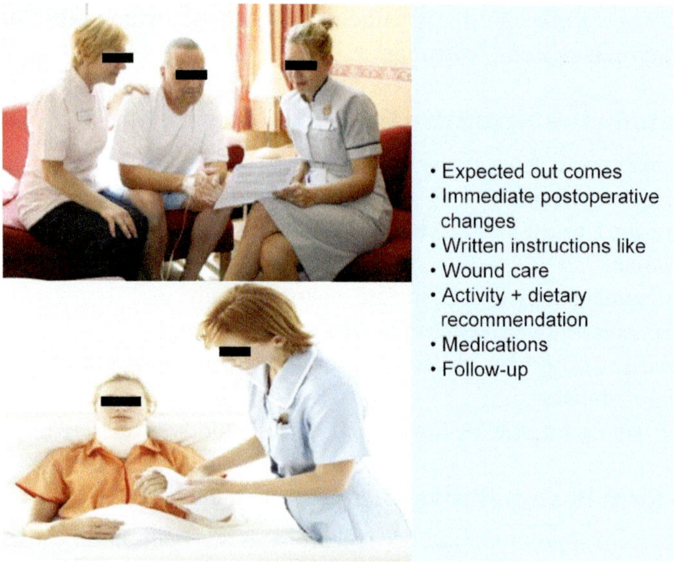

Fig. 5: Teaching, patient self care.

- *Bleeding:* Immediate medical attention needed if heavy bleeding or prolonged spotting occurs.
- Hematoma at the surgery site
- *Urinary retention:* Pay attention to difficulty urination or incomplete emptying of the bladder.[4]
- *Wound dehiscence:* Be watchful
- Pulmonary embolism
- Septicemia

Tips for a Smooth Recovery to the Patient

- Patients should follow healthcare provider instructions. Adhere to postoperative instructions **(Fig. 5)**.
- *Rest:* Avoid overexertion and prioritize rest
- *Stay hydrated:* Advice to drink plenty of fluids
- *Seek support:* whenever necessary.
- Monitor for complications and seek medical attention promptly

Postoperative Nursing Care

- Avoid coughing, sneezing straining because these increase intraocular pressure.[8]
- Assess for postoperative pain—approach from unaffected side
- Assess for surgical complications
- *Teach home care:*

- Timely medicines intake
- Knowledge about symptoms to report
- Photophobia

CONCLUSION

Postoperative care in vaginal surgery is crucial for a successful recovery. By following these guidelines and attending follow-up appointments, patients can minimize complications and ensure a smooth transition back to normal activities. Healthcare providers play a vital role in educating patients on postoperative care and monitoring their progress.

Benefits of Postoperative Care

- A speedy recovery
- A better quality of life
- By better postoperative care, there are less chance of negative side effects and health issues.
- Patient regains early control of personal and professional things
- Postoperative care gives patient sense of well-being.

REFERENCES

1. Nelson G, Altman AD, Nick A, Meyer LA, Ramirez PT, Achtari C, et al. Guidelines for pre- and intra-operative care in gynecologic/oncology surgery: Enhanced Recovery After Surgery (ERAS®) Society recommendations. Gynecol Oncol. 2015 doi: 10.1016/j.ygyno.2015.11.015. [PubMed] [CrossRef].
2. Gustafsson UO, Scott MJ, Schwenk W, Demartines N, Roulin D, Francis N, et al. Guidelines for perioperative care in elective colonic surgery: enhanced recovery after surgery (ERAS) society recommendations. World J Surg. 2012;37(2):259-84. [PubMed] [Google Scholar]
3. Nygren J, Thacker J, Carli F, Fearon KC, Norderval S, Lobo DN, et al. Guidelines for perioperative care in elective rectal/pelvic surgery: Enhanced Recovery After Surgery (ERAS) Society recommendations. World J Surg. 2013;37(2):285-305. [PubMed] [Google Scholar]
4. Guyatt GH, Oxman AD, Vist GE, Kunz R, Falck-Ytter Y, Alonso-Coello P, et al. GRADE: an emerging consensus on rating quality of evidence and strength of recommendations. BMJ. 2008;336(7650):924-6. [PMC free article] [PubMed] [Google Scholar]
5. Cerantola Y, Valerio M, Persson B, Jichlinski P, Ljungqvist O, Hubner M, et al. Guidelines for perioperative care after radical cystectomy for bladder cancer: enhanced recovery after surgery (ERAS®) Society recommendations. Clin Nutr. 2013;32(6):879-87. [PubMed] [Google Scholar]
6. Brunetti M, Shemilt I, Pregno S, Vale L, Oxman AD, Lord J, et al. GRADE guidelines: 10. Considering resource use and rating the quality of economic evidence. J Clin Epidemiol. 2013;66(2):140-50. [PubMed] [Google Scholar]
7. Clarke-Pearson DL, Synan IS, Dodge R, Soper JT, Berchuck A, Coleman RE. A randomized trial of low-dose heparin and intermittent pneumatic calf

compression for the prevention of deep venous thrombosis after gynecologic oncology surgery. Am J Obstet Gynecol. 1993;168(4):1146-53. (discussion 1153-4) [PubMed] [Google Scholar]

8. Maxwell GL, Synan I, Dodge R, Carroll B, Clarke-Pearson DL. Pneumatic compression versus low molecular weight heparin in gynecologic oncology surgery: a randomized trial. Obstet Gynecol. 2001;98(6):989-95. [PubMed] [Google Scholar]
9. Einstein MH, Kushner DM, Connor JP, Bohl AA, Best TJ, Evans MD, et al. A protocol of dual prophylaxis for venous thromboembolism prevention in gynecologic cancer patients. Obstet Gynecol. 2008;112(5):1091-7. [PubMed] [Google Scholar]
10. Sachdeva A, Dalton M, Amaragiri SV, Lees T. Graduated compression stockings for prevention of deep vein thrombosis. Cochrane Database Syst Rev. 2014;12:CD001484. [PubMed] [Google Scholar]